THE UNSEEN WISDOM OF THE UNBORN

Is your future decided before birth?

Atul K. Mehra

Published by Mehra Publishers
Toronto, Canada

Ordering Information:
Quantity sales. Special discounts are available on quantity purchases by corporations, associations, and others. Printed in the **Canada**.

Library of Congress Control Number: 2017956542 (First Edition)

Second Edition
ISBN-13: 979-86655179-1-9 Paperback
ISBN-13: 978-1-7772753-1-0 eBook

First Edition
ISBN-13:   Softcover   978-1-64069-736-2
            Pdf   978-1-64069-737-9
            ePub   978-1-64069-738-6
            Kindle   978-1-64069-739-3

Rev. date: 06/30/2020

THE UNSEEN WISDOM OF THE UNBORN

This book is dedicated

To the loving memory of my father, Raghu Nath Mehra
and also to my mother, Darshi Mehra

About the Author

Atul Kumar Mehra is an author, international speaker and a Registered Psychotherapist in Ontario, Canada. He has participated in Moderated Panel Discussion Videos with Dr. John Gray (The author of *Women are from Venus and Men are from Mars*) on various topics. He has been a guest speaker on hundreds of TV and radio shows in different languages, as well as a keynote presenter for national and international conferences.

Atul was born in New Delhi, India, and obtained a Masters' degree in India and in Integrative Therapy of Depth Psychology from Germany. He now resides in Mississauga, Ontario, Canada, with his wife and two daughters.

Atul has always had a love of writing and has published articles in several countries and in several languages. In addition to this book, he is also working on two other books - *Addiction is Survival, Not Guilt* and *How to Program your Subconscious Mind.*

When he isn't working, Atul enjoys playing chess, reading and writing. He also teaches yoga, meditation and dancing meditation and is a huge football fan. He loves to travel and meet people, and is fluent in Spanish, English, Hindi, and Punjabi. He has done voluntary work with senior citizens in Venezuela.

In the future, Atul will continue writing additional books, to share his knowledge with a wide cross-section of people, and to enjoy the love and company of his family.

You can keep up with Atul Kumar Mehra at www.atulmehra.com

Contents

Acknowledgements

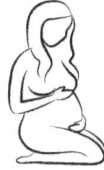

No mother is bad otherwise we would not be here. I always relate this sentence as a response whenever I hear someone criticizing or speaking unkindly of their mother. I cannot help but think that our parents did their very best in raising us, given the time period and their circumstances. And, we will do the very same for our children.

So, in that vein, I would like to dedicate this book first and foremost to my mother, Darshi Mehra, and my late father, Raghu Nath Mehra, both of whom were my very first teachers in life, and who accepted and allowed me to be who I am. Their love, appreciation, and faith guided and encouraged me through every step in my life, even when I hit rock bottom several times. I am also very grateful to my late grandmother, Raj Mehra, who spoke to my mother about the experience of the mother's womb when my mother was carrying my younger brother. It was this event that ignited a curiosity in me about the mysterious life growing inside the womb – a curiosity that culminated in this book. I would also like to extend my gratitude to my late grandparents, Jagat Ram Mehra and Raj Mehra, Moti Ram and my grandmother Dulari Kapoor, who have always loved me unconditionally.

This book would not be a reality without my lovely and loving wife, Tatiana Mehra, who is a very important and indispensable part of my life. Not only has she encouraged, loved and supported me through its every page and every moment, but also has blessed me with two beautiful daughters, Anisha Mehra and Ambar

Mehra. Both of my loving daughters bring me immeasurable joy and have gifted me my life's purpose, allowing me to relive those glorious days of intrauterine experiences or "seeds" that germinated into ideas and discoveries contained within this book.

My gratitude also extends to my supportive siblings, Rinku Mehra and Abhinav Mehra, who have accompanied and helped me whenever I needed them the most. They have always been there for me through all sorts of experiences in my life.

I would also like to take this opportunity to thank everyone who has been part of my life all these years, and has influenced me during my childhood in one way or another. Among them are my family members: Shyam, Bholi, Santosh, Tinku, Buna, and Deepak. A very special mention to Arturo, Martha, Mauricio and especially to Maruja Calderorn, as well as to Anchal, Pooja and Ariv.

I extend my sincere gratitude to my dearest friends and teachers, Werner Meinhold and Jose Villalba, both of whom encouraged me to journey into the depths of psychology to reveal and understand the unconscious levels so that I could unravel the mysteries and secrets of a mother-to-be and her unborn baby.

I am also grateful to all my clients, in particular to Rosio Galarza, who helped me navigate into the depths of the unconscious mind in order to reveal the deepest, hidden secrets of the Self that reside within our psyche.

This book would not be complete without a special mention of my friends, Kristy Higgins and Dinesh Bharuchi, whose constant encouragement and belief in my work propelled me forward to write this book.

My sincere thanks extends to two special people who helped me with the completion of my book. My sincere thanks goes to Anjana Thom, who helped me by editing this book with patience and understanding, and has also provided valuable feedback in finalizing the title of the book. My heartfelt and deepest thanks also to my wonderfully creative and generous brother-in-law, David Arias, who diligently donated his time and expertise in creating a beautiful cover for my book.

Above all else, I am eternally grateful to God, whose divine love and spiritual guidance inspired me to actualize this book and to make this day possible.

Foreword

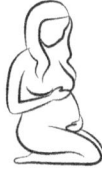

My friend, Atul Mehra, a renowned Psychotherapist and learned author of this book titled, *The Unseen Wisdom of the Unborn*, shares a wonderful spiritual and professional relationship with me. As an ardent researcher of depth psychology, Atul has packed an unbelievable amount of information in this book.

By the virtue of his subjective experiences and case studies, Atul has very lucidly and powerfully combined spiritual and psychological concepts to introduce an entirely new concept of holism that is a positive and soul-enriching experience.

The effort is to balance the travails of a new, upcoming life (Unborn Child) with a peaceful and positive experience. This experience is the fulfillment of a woman who is going to become a mother. She, on her behalf, needs to be guided by a positive mindset that reflects an element of contentment and satisfaction, forgiveness, and originality, love and courage.

The outcome of this is most priceless -- a child born of and with wisdom!

Without going into every detail that the author has delved in, I am confident that this book is meant for every reader who wishes to undertake a quest for unravelling the secret behind the womb awakening - the cradle of conscious positive transformation.

Dr. R.K. Raina
New Delhi, India
On Wednesday, February 8, 2017

Mother is an essence, baby is an existence,
And together they celebrate God's creation.
Atul Mehra

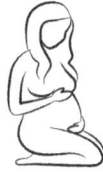

Introduction

Not many books have been written on the topic of intrauterine life. Our modern world considers the beginning of life to be when a baby is born of its mother's womb. The intrauterine life has been of very little or no significance to many of us. An historical Sanskrit epic in India named "Mahabharata" speaks of how as an unborn child in his mother's womb, Abhimanyu, learns how to breach a seemingly impenetrable and complex concentric defense formation. The epic explains that he overhears his father talking to his mother about the importance of this defensive strategy while he was still in the womb, and how to enter it and stay safe in order to defeat one's enemies. This bit of information later plays a very significant role during the epic battle, enabling Abhimanyu to breach the defense formation and overcome many of his foes.

I remember a time as a young boy when my Mom was pregnant with my younger brother, my grandmother Raj Mehra counselled her not to watch any negative movies or read any negative materials. She encouraged my mother to dedicate her time listening to good music and performing prayers to God. According to my grandmother, the mother's thoughts – positive or negative – directly impact the baby's personality. I could not understand this at that time. However, after several years of treating many patients, it was confirmed to me that their parent's thoughts had affected their lives. It was really amazing to me that my Grandmother and her generation were privy to this important piece of knowledge.

From then on my curiosity took root, and from it grew many shoots, and soon it grew into something bigger and stronger. Although I had lived a healthy intrauterine life, my experience as a practitioner working with my clients made it necessary for me to write this book to make these ideas explicit. In fact, this idea has transformed itself into something quite symbolic for me.

As individuals we continue to evolve spiritually and psychologically, as a race we continue to make scientific and social progress, but collectively, we remain in the dark about the secret life of the unborn. The research on intrauterine life has rejected a lot of scepticism. Today, we know that in the second trimester of pregnancy, the foetus can recognize sounds and smells, and in the sixth month it can perceive light. Despite this knowledge, the idea that a foetus could have emerging awareness, awakening senses, and memories of living in its mother's womb is still doubted or denied in many circles today. To understand this, we need to go beyond analytical thoughts and judgements and draw from the truths that exist within our own frame of reference and way of thinking.

I propose that you undertake a journey into the unknown with me. Just be ready to navigate the pages of this book carefully through the summarized histories of my clients so that you may experience being in a new dimension, different than anything you have ever experienced.

In this book, I will present different yet exceptional evidences gathered from my years of research working with different people. These people have allowed me, during their therapeutic process, to glimpse into their intrauterine memories as they relived those experiences. Through these accounts we will take a look at the deepest mysteries hidden inside a tiny being that is still growing in its mother's womb.

The intrauterine life is the life beyond space and time, although ironically, it exists in space and time. Not only does the baby record external information (i.e. visual, auditory impressions), but it also experiences internal emotions such as rejection and love. These impressions do not have an analytical language but in fact, they have a language of their own in the form of images, sounds, and emotions; and strangely enough, they are the foundation for attracting the rest of life experiences. They are like footprints that are permanently etched in our unconscious minds that can only be retraced or accessed in a special relaxation state, enabling us to understand how we can live our life as a "whole."

This is the time when we must perceive and not attempt to explain or understand. If we are to have a conversation about the bond of love between a baby and its parents, then it is time to think outside the box and allow ourselves to understand those gentle messages of the intrauterine life that have made such a wonderful connection possible.

Each one of us has the ability and skills to shape our lives into something beautiful and joyful. You can abandon that painful mask of anguish and connect with your inner self *only if you want to*. The pages in this book serve as a guide to show you how to break free from negative patterns and reconnect with positive ones. If you are seeking to transform some things in your life, then this book will communicate those key messages you need in order to make it happen.

At this present time, after having facilitated more than 7,000 sessions, I am ready to share this information with you. My vocation to be the "Researcher of the Unconscious" has come to fruition as each passing day strengthens my conviction about the importance of intrauterine life, of the foetus, and of the future birth of a human.

Many thanks go to my teachers and clients who have contributed directly or indirectly to this book. Now all parents can better understand the connection between different emotions and "thinking patterns" of their babies and the circumstances they may later encounter. This will help them to create a positive and loving narrative with the baby so that they may establish a closer relationship from the first instance.

Once a client remarked to me that if pregnant moms were to undertake this therapy, then they would prevent many future traumas and problems from happening in their children's lives. To add to that observation, I would like to emphasize that not only would the future moms benefit from this therapy, but also each one of us.

Atul Kumar Mehra

"Correct" is a dream.
"False" is also a dream.
Master Takuan

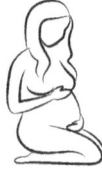

Chapter 1

Hypnosis and Intrauterine Life

The word 'hypnosis' is derived from the Greek word *Hypnos*, which is often considered as sleep as well as death. In Greek mythology, in fact, Hypnos and Thanatos are twin brothers, with Thanatos being the God of Death and Hypnos being the God of Sleep.

When we hear the word Hypnosis, we imagine ourselves being under the command of another who orders us to do some ridiculous thing or another; or, we imagine ourselves giving up control to the hypnotist who then manipulates us to say or do things against our will. Others may hold an opinion that under hypnosis, the client is in an unconscious state and therefore, unaware of what is happening. Some may even think that the state of hypnosis is an altered state of consciousness. Some consider hypnosis as a suggestive therapy. We might even feel fearful about being hypnotized; yet at the same time, our curiosity gets the better of us. Could it be said that you do not know what is happening around you when you are in hypnosis?

Honestly, none of the above statements are true. Nobody can hypnotize you. Perhaps when you reach a stage in hypnosis – a kind of Somnambulism Hypnosis – that possibly could happen. However, you can only reach that stage if you allow, by your free will, the hypnotist to guide you there, and then offer no resistance when instructions are given to you. Of course, Somnambulism Hypnosis has helped many people in certain ways, however, from the perspective of Depth Psychology, it is said that these instances can be the repetition of a symbolic domineering father who makes his son obey. In order to be accepted by his symbolic father, the obedient son then humbly follows instructions. This can repeat and reinforce the childhood traumas at a subconscious level.

Surprisingly, about 95% of our life is lived under hypnosis, using a mere 5% in a state of vigilance—when we engage in an affair, an addiction, a phobia, or are in conflict with someone, an inability to control our emotions, psychological or emotional dependency etc. Honestly, how many times have we have tried to be sad or depressed rationally or knowingly in our life?

In hypnosis you do not sleep nor do you lose your consciousness; it is simply a deep state of concentration in which the person is even more awake than before. Thus, it cannot be considered as an altered state of consciousness. Rather, it is a natural, basic and a very special type of an inner awareness or sensitivity.

In our daily activities we use a state of vigilance interspersed with hypnotic state as many of these activities are performed unconsciously. This means that there is never 100% vigilance. For example, when we watch a movie, we know that it is a fictional drama, nevertheless we become hypnotized as our emotions pull us into feeling sad, happy or scared based on the scenes before us. There is a state of vigilance and hypnosis present simultaneously. Another example is when we sleep and have a dream, but then we remember some of that dream. In that, there is a mixture of sleep and vigilance. Everybody experiences a state of hypnosis in his or her daily life.

The old definition of *hypnosis* is currently used to denote a phenomenon of the so-called "third state of consciousness," just the same as a *state of vigilance* (first state) and as a *dream* (second state). It is commonly understood as an "extraordinary" state of limited consciousness, close to a dream.

According to the new definition coined by Werner Meinhold, hypnosis is the first state of consciousness. He explains that "hypnosis" is neither a dream nor an "extraordinary" state. Rather it consists of several states of consciousness that are very natural as they correspond to the archaic structures of the brain and their specific functions. Following are the foremost structures of the brain:

a) The right hemisphere of the cortex
b) The Limbic system
c) The Stem

These archaic structures with their functions accompany and influence us all in our daily lives in a continuous and indispensable way, and yet they remain at an unconscious level. Under conscious hypnosis, these processes can be recognized due to the fact that several hypnotic states of consciousness (the states during the evolution of Central Nervous System as mentioned in the chapter Mammalian vs. Reptilian consciousness) are evolutionarily older ones. At the same time, they are the basis for other vital functions and states of consciousness. Meinhold called hypnosis the "first state of consciousness".

In order to better understand their function in everyday life, I will use an example. For example, you are driving a car and somebody appears in front of you out of nowhere; you immediately hit the brake pedal as an automatic response. This is triggered within the right hemisphere or the archaic structure of brain, which reacts to and registers your anxiety and fear caused by your perception of danger or threat from this event. Now, it takes some time for the left hemisphere or the rational part of the brain to enter the scene; maybe somebody near you says, "Thank God, nothing happened and now you can calm down." Your anxiety and fear may have appeared instantaneously, but it will take a longer time to calm down. The anxiety response is triggered by the limbic system, which is located in the right hemisphere, or the archaic brain.

On the other hand, the slower process of rationalization corresponds to the new brain or the Neocortex. The information that is communicated from the "old brain" is much faster than the information communicated from the "new brain". This is why we quickly arouse to anger, but we are slower to calm down. We always live in this fight zone throughout our lives. When we perform an action based on emotions then we could say that we have done something irrational; conversely, if we do something rational we could say that we have suppressed our emotions. The fight between these two hemispheres is like the battle of the Titans. We need to learn how to create a balance between the two zones so we may create a healthy life for ourselves. That can be done when we begin to use our sense of awareness in everything we do in our daily lives.

Hypnosis remains the predominant state of consciousness until the age of 6 or 7, after which the cortex begins to influence and dominate the child's consciousness. This is also the time when a child begins elementary school. From conception until the first 3 years of its life, a baby lives in a deep state of hypnosis and is unable to differentiate between reality and fantasy. For example, your first language is English and you learn it naturally from your parents. You do not challenge them for the way they teach you to speak or to understand English. However, as you get older – say, around 15 years old or even earlier – you begin to realize that you speak English. Later on, you may choose to learn a new language such as German or Italian. You will then use English as the basis for learning this new language, and you may begin to actively discuss the significance of certain English words.

The first man in your life was your father and the first woman in your life was your mother (generally speaking where all other situations remain equal). From conception until the first 3 years of your life, the impressions, experiences, and events – seen, heard, imagined, and experienced – become the basis of your personality and throughout your life you will continue to attract and be influenced by life experiences based on that.

Two-year-olds cannot rationalize as an adult can. It is almost impossible to explain to a two year-old child that her father cannot afford to buy her the doll that she is so desperate to have. It is also not advisable for young children to watch violent TV programs or be exposed to parental conflicts, arguments or other unhealthy and negative experiences because they are most likely to show aggressive behaviour and to view the world as a scary place.

Living in a constant state of awareness is key to emerging from our hypnotic state. In India, the word *maya* is used to denote this state. I consider *maya* and *hypnosis* to be one and the same. *Maya* in Hindi means ignorance or illusion. We regard ourselves as the proud owners of possessions such as cars, houses, electronics, jewellery, etc. We spend thousands of dollars to look our best, or to have a great figure, whether it is through plastic surgery or gym memberships. I am not saying that these are wrong or that you should not enjoy your possessions. However, when they start dominating your life and become the reason to live, it is then that suffering and ignorance usually ensue. This is the state that I refer to as *maya* – ignorance or hypnosis. We live a hypnotic life when we are slaves to material objects and our success is dependent upon how much wealth or status we have amassed. The richer and more famous we are, the more importance we are given. That is supreme ignorance because it fails to consider that the only reality in life is death and everything else is simply a possibility. Death is the great equalizer – rich or poor, beautiful or ugly, famous or forgotten. The perception of material possessions as belonging to me is merely temporary and hypnotic. If we detach ourselves from these limiting and illusory perceptions, then we evolve into higher levels of consciousness. Emerging from that level of ignorance is the same as becoming independent of *maya*. Life is a complete set of different experiences at different ages and stages; everything that "belongs" to us today may belong to someone else tomorrow. Isn't that amazing?

This research offers a new paradigm of science, which states that by adopting a holistic vision we can establish that in the utero phase there is a very deep attachment to the psychic and spiritual levels, both of which supersede the biological level. Hypnosis is a natural state of consciousness up until school age because the cortex does not begin to dominate the consciousness until then. Further to this connection, the pregnant mom-to-be's attitude towards the child in her womb becomes the main source of health and happiness or misery and disease in her child.

Science is continuously transforming and evolving, while the development of new technologies has resulted in creating excellent research systems. As science evolves, it postulates new theories to understand the world, constructs new realities and seeks new possibilities, while discarding the old and worn out viewpoints that no longer fit the paradigm.

The understanding of psychic union between the child and the mother in the utero phase introduces us to a new organic-spiritual paradigm, which goes beyond the limited and materialistic world view of the Cartesian paradigm (reason and feeling are separate; matter and spirit are not the same).

This chapter takes us on a journey from the mechanistic to the holistic paradigm.

*The genesis of the world is a psychic act
and from this self-recognition originates the
evolution of the physical world.*
Mircea Eliade (From the Hindu wisdom)

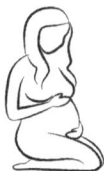

Chapter 2

Reptilian Consciousness vs. Mammalian Consciousness

The Evolution of Central Nervous System

Our brain is an astonishing wonder designed by Mother Nature. Imagine, hundreds of billions of cells creating 100 trillion connections, billions of signals interconnecting and making us who we are. This small yet amazing container with a jelly-like mass and weighing approximately 3 pounds has been creating a plethora of questions and puzzling many scientists, researchers, and meditation practitioners alike.

It is really interesting to understand the history of the evolution of the human mind. How did it all begin? What were the first evolutionary steps or changes that took place hundreds of millions of years ago? Although many years of research and investigation have gone into understanding the simple yet complex functions of our brain, it still remains a challenge to understand its origins of the human mind and its maximum functioning capacity.

The human brain contains over 11 billion specialized nerve cells, or neurons, capable of receiving, processing, and relaying the electrochemical pulses upon which all our sensations, imagination, actions, thoughts, and emotions rest; but the most exciting part is not only the sheer number of neurons alone, but also how they are organized and interconnected.

The evolutionary history of each part of our Central Nervous System (CNS) allows us to draw an important conclusion for the understanding of the human nature and its development. According to scientific research, the human brain has undergone a very complex evolution for nearly 3.8 million years. Starting from unicellular consciousness, the human brain evolved in several stages: cellular colony consciousness - multicellular consciousness - nervous system - reptilian consciousness - mammalian consciousness - primate consciousness - primitive consciousness - left hemisphere/logical-analytical consciousness which is only 30,000 years to 5,000 years old. *

It is important to mention here that the Biogenetics law (theory of development) of HAECKEL. It is a theory in biology by a German atheist and zoologist Ernest Haeckel. It indicates that every childhood is a natural hypnosis, suggesting that the ontogenesis (individual development) repeats the phylogenesis (group development). This is why every human undergoes the complete evolution process of the human brain during his or her embryonic and child development. It begins with a primary cell, passing through the archaic structures with their corresponding states of hypnotic consciousness to culminate with the most

*The development stages of the Central Nervous System have been written in its simplest form to explain the evolution of a baby in the mother's womb and they may differ from other reports available; nevertheless, they maintain their essence about development of consciousness.

developed awareness of the left hemisphere of the cortex. It is only 30,000 to 5,000 years old – also known as neocortex or cerebral cortex – and is considered as wakefulness, the seat of self-consciousness, or the logic-rational centre of the brain.

Although this law is criticized and discredited by many, several observers have noted various connections between phylogeny and ontogeny, explaining them in terms of evolutionary theory and taking them as supporting evidence for the theory. For example, the backbone – a common structure among all vertebrates – appears as one of the earliest structures laid out in all vertebrate embryos. Research in the late 20th century confirmed that "both biological evolution and the stages in the child's cognitive development follow much the same progression of evolutionary stages as that suggested in the archaeological record (Wikipedia). I do not want to go into further complicated details of biogenetic law's veracity; my only idea is to use it as a reference in order to explain the importance of mammalian and reptilian consciousness, as both have played a significant and interesting role in the lives of my clients struggling with abandonment issues.

OUR OLD AND THE NEW BRAIN

Mother Nature is characterized by love, glue that binds us all together. This is the same that happens to our consciousness as well. Our brain has several different areas that evolved at different times. When an area in our ancestor's brain grew it was not discarded, but retained by nature and rather it transformed into the most recent newer level. Today, the cerebral cortex/neocortex is considered as a new and important area of the human brain, covering and including the oldest, most primitive parts. These primitive regions have not been eliminated, but rather they remain active while staying "invisible", and hold an undisputed control over the human body. These primitive parts of the human brain continue to operate in accordance with a stereotyped and instinctive set of programs that come from mammals and from an older species of reptiles that gave rise to the mammalian tribe.

Experiments have shown that a large part of human behaviour originates from the areas of the brain that once controlled the vital actions of our ancestors but now remains deeply buried. Now, let us take an example, reptiles have three main basic functions: hunger, sleep and survival, including the flight or fight response.

Imagine that you are in a place where you are witnessing beautiful teachings of non violence, respect and courtesy. Out of nowhere somebody screams "F...i...re!!!!!" More than likely, you will get nervous as you see others running for the door. You quickly forget those logical and respectful scenes you just witnessed, and do not hesitate to step on others to save your own life. This proves the undisputed control of our body by our primitive reptilian brain, which is concerned solely with survival.

How hard would it be for us to imagine a group of parents who never take care of their offspring? As soon as they give birth to their young, the parents abandon them, not feeling any remorse, guilt or regret in doing so. What if the 'watching over pattern' never existed in their brain and abandonment was their natural reaction? Would you blame them for abandoning their babies? What would happen to their babies? Would they survive or die? If they manage to survive, then how would their adult lives turn out?

The reptilian brain is responsible for survival instincts. Reptiles do not protect their hatchlings. On occasion, the young hatchlings may become a tasty snack for the parent, and in some cases they are completely abandoned and left to fend for themselves. The young reptiles fight for survival, so they come into this world equipped with all the necessary programming imprinted on their brains. They are like miniature adults from the moment they take birth.

Then, millions of year later, reptiles started evolving and the first mammals were formed. The most important part of mammalian nature was the parental care of its offspring. The little, helpless baby mammals needed parental care for survival. Over many generations, parental indifference traits were eliminated and all adult mammals that survived in the wild became caring and attentive parents. To accommodate this new form of behaviour, new programs were encoded into the human brain. New parts of mammalian consciousness were fused with those of reptilian consciousness. Along with the old programs of hunger, sleep and survival, there were new added responsibilities of parental care and protection. Both primitive and mammalian brain regions are completely wrapped and buried under the cerebral cortex, but they continue to exert a great deal of unseen influence and control over many of our everyday actions and behaviours.

It is a little bit easier to understand when we witness such types of abandonment cases. The reptilian part of our brain would have been more active at the time of abandonment but when we feel guilty about not taking care of our children, we are doing so from the mammalian consciousness part of our brain. The mammalian brain is responsible for feeling and memory.

In order to give more weight to this discovery with my clients, I was looking for more scientific-based evidence, and as luck would have it, I came across an online article that appeared in a newspaper named "The Tuscaloosa News," printed on Dec. 6, 1981. The famous author Dr. Robert Jastraw, an internationally known astronomer and authority on life in the cosmos wrote:

"Experiments suggest that parental feelings source of some of the finest emotions still originate in these primitive programmed areas of the brain that go back to the time of

old Mammal more than 100 million years ago. In one experiment the cerebral cortex was removed from the brain of a female hamster, leaving only the reptile and old-mammal center of instinctive behavior. Yet the small hamster matured normally, showed an interest in male hamsters, gave birth and was a good mother. It still retained "hamster nature - the equivalent of human nature."

In another experiment, only the ancient mammalian center of instinctive behavior was removed and the female hamster lost all interest in caring for her newborns. How intriguing!

A very important part of the primitive brain – the size of a walnut – is known as the *hypothalamus* that forms a part of the limbic system. It controls body temperature, hunger, thirst, fatigue, sleep and important parts of parenting and attachment behavior. An electrical stimulus applied to a particular part of hypothalamus for a short period of time in the brain of any mammal or a human can trigger the emotional state of anxiety, anger, fear, and other negative feelings.

It is incredible to know more that there are two separate "minds" residing in one body. One is ruled by emotions that has evolved over millions of years and contains ancient consciousness such as the reptilian and the mammalian. The second mind is ruled by reason and resides in the cerebral cortex. Generally, the new brain masters the old brain. For example, we live our daily lives with analytical reasoning, but when we feel anger or fear, we may go into what we call as an "out of control" state because our emotions can override reason. If an angry person becomes mindful of his anger, then he can witness it but still may be unable to stop. He may feel divided into two separate parts and feel that his center is no longer in his body. Even if someone were to try to calm him down with reason, it would take some time.

The information coming from the old brain for action is faster than the new brain. For example, it is an automatic old brain response to feel panic and anxiety, such as when we hit the brake pedal when someone unexpectedly cuts in front of our car (emotions). It takes some time to calm down after the ordeal is over (reason).

Now we can understand the magnitude of processes taking place in our brain that enable us to feel and live a variety of emotions such as love, fear, anger, joy, hate, guilt, affection, etc. How are these emotions created? How are difficult experiences lived by the mother during pregnancy perceived by the baby? How can it affect the rest of his life? The baby, from the time of conception to almost up to three years of age, just experiences and lives in the emotional brain. He cannot rationally understand what his mother feels, nor is he concerned with what is right or wrong. If his mother had continuous traumatic experiences, sending painful signals to the emotional brain, she is likely to live with more anxiety, depression, fear or anger. Her baby will find this as the only way to connect with his mother and will seek similar kinds of difficult experiences, generally attracting such situations in adult life. This is often an unconscious form of connecting with his mother.

Feelings are part of the emotional brain and are deeply rooted in the inner recesses of our mind. Although there have been some interesting discoveries, there is still a great deal more to research and to understand. All of the experiences lived during pregnancy become the base of our emotional responses in our life. All modern diseases of emotional, physical, mental, or spiritual nature originate as seeds in the mother's womb. Surprisingly enough, there are effective techniques such as "Integrative in-depth psychology therapy" developed by Werner Meinhold that go beyond different modern methods and into the realms where one becomes aware of these processes as a means to treat physical and mental disorders.

Our mind is comprised of various stages of evolution of the central nervous system, including the emotional and the rational brain. Its scientifically proven properties continually lead us on a journey to its advancement. As evolution progresses, the human brain continues to grow new layers over the old ones; who knows, the next stage of brain evolution will witness a new and enhanced brain being formed over the present cerebral cortex, paving the way for a superior way of life.

At bottom, the ordinary is not ordinary;
it is extraordinary
Martin Heidegger

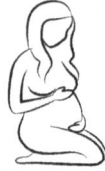

Chapter 3

Does Spermatozoon have Consciousness?

Sperm is the male reproductive cell in vertebrates. The term is derived from Latin word *sperma* meaning seed or semen, and from the Greek word *sperma* meaning seed of plants and animals. Does the sperm have consciousness? Does it think thoughts, feel emotions, or have any sentiments? How does it know where to travel? How does it know where its destination lies? Does it feel happy or sad? These are the many curious questions that arise when we begin to ponder the importance of the microscopic and oft-forgotten spermatozoon.

Many years ago when I was in a session with one of my clients, she started asking questions about the sperm, spermatozoon and other forms of words used during conception and pregnancy. I explained the significance of these words to her; and that was the moment when I decided that were I to write an article or chapter on this topic, I would explain the differences and provide more information about the sperm. Hence, now I have used the word Spermatozoon in the title of this chapter, instead of the word Sperm. Immediately after that thought, another thought occurred to me, which gave me cause for a good laugh: *"Thank God, the sperm does not have to change or remember all these names or nouns during the whole process otherwise it might get confused and end up somewhere else."*

My curiosity about the sperm's life grew more after I lived those moments of sperm-consciousness in my own life while I was undergoing Whole Life Therapy. This therapeutic process was part of my training that led to me obtaining my specialized diploma as a practitioner of Integrative Therapy of Depth Psychology under the expert guidance of my supervisor and friend, Dr. Jose Villalba, a clinical Psychologist. Although I found it extremely interesting, I could not believe it at that time. I thought of it as a part of my active imagination; however, that mindfulness of a singular cell consciousness I experienced completely amazed and surprised me. During those moments I could "feel" and "live" the information I was carrying as an accepted child; that sensation and perception of being happy and satisfied and moving fast among so many other sperm was beyond any reasoning and imagination. The moments of consciousness I lived as a sperm cannot be verified or defined by current scientific facts or research. I may be able to describe the experiences in words but living the moments defies my intellectual reasoning and lies beyond my imagination.

Although I felt and lived those moments so intensely, I began to doubt myself for many days afterwards. Soon after, I began working my clients who lived and described the moments of sperm consciousness. They were able to analyze and understand the impact of these experiences in their daily life. This brought me to a point where I was able to replace doubt with faith.

Since a majority of my clients have had very similar encounters, I was able to connect with them on a deeper level. Each time a client described his experience while in session, I was able to connect with what they were describing and help them dissolve the feelings and issues around malignant impregnations. I was surprised at how it was possible for me to feel those sensations even though they were experienced and described by my clients. Later, while doing a demonstration in front of some students, I realized that the connection I had with my clients was due to my earlier experience of my therapy process, which helped me to relive the psycho-spiritual state many times over. Connecting with those sensations still sometimes gives me a kind of spiritual shivering.

While conducting research, I found similar experiences lived by Dr. Graham Farrent, an Australian psychiatrist, who against all his clinical training emphasized the importance of Cellular Consciousness and Conception. During his visit to the U.S.A., he gave an interview in which he shared his experiences of a pre-conception consciousness during a primal therapy session. I thought it is useful to include this information because it might substantiate the experience for my dear readers and help them to develop a better understanding of this topic.

Now, moving ahead with all this information, it is time for us to understand and appreciate a little bit more about this little astonishing seed that carries the promise of a great life ahead.

Nature maintains its balance in all aspects of life. All living things are made up of cells whether it is a plant, an animal or a human. Those that are made of one cell are known as unicellular organisms. Others that are made from a large number of cells are known as multicellular organisms. Cells are so tiny that they are invisible to the naked eye; they can only be seen through a microscope. Each cell in our body is made from an already existing cell. According to the researchers, our body replaces itself with a new set of cells every seven to ten years. Each cell is suited with the size and shape it needs in order to do its assigned job. These cells combine together to form tissues such as muscles, skin, bones, and organs.

In a cellular life cycle, every cell gives birth to two identical daughter-cells, a process known as *mitosis*. The main purpose of mitosis is to reproduce new cells for growth and to repair aging and damaged tissues throughout our bodies. This is opposed to the process of sexual reproduction, known as *meiosis,* where a cell gives birth to four daughter-cells.

Each human cell contains 23 pairs of chromosomes. In simple terms, a chromosome can be described as a nucleus of a living cell, which carries genetic information in the form of genes and transmits hereditary information. The semen is a generative substance from the father that carries a unicellular organism or a single cell known as the sperm. Semen is alkaline and does not allow the sperm to be completely motile until it reaches the female reproductive tract. A non-motile sperm is *spermatium* and a motile sperm is known as *spermatozoon*, the reproductive cell or gamete of the male. It combines with the gamete of the female known as an ovum to form a zygote, which marks the beginning of a new life. This zygote-formation process is called "fertilization" or "conception" where twenty-three father chromosomes join with twenty-three mother chromosomes. This is a moment in time when the soul descends into a newly-formed body.

The stage before conception is considered as prenatal. The embryo is the developing pregnancy from the time of fertilization until the eighth week. From eight weeks until the moment of birth the embryo develops as a foetus. The process of development in the uterus from conception to birth is also known as gestation.

By using layman's language and cutting through unnecessary scientific jargon, I hope that I have helped you to understand the reproduction process in its simplest form even though this information is easily accessible everywhere. Isn't it better to read this information in an easy-to-understand way in one place?

Considering all the experiences we live in the various stages of our lives, we can say that we have a cellular memory (sperm), egg memory, a soul memory, conception memory, embryo memory, or foetus memory, moments before and after the birth memory. As we live the moments in our lives, these experiences become an integral part of our memory and of our cellular consciousness.

Present-day scientific community is reluctant to accept the existence of cellular consciousness. Even after many years of scientific research and evidence gathering, scientists refuse to accept the possibility that deeper truths reside at the cellular level. One could accept these assertions at their face value, or have a session where one could possibly experience his/her life as sperm-consciousness and then use this powerful information to heal any current disorders and diseases that seem resistant to treatment.

We know that every cell in our body has consciousness. The cell is the basic structural and functional unit of all known living organisms. It is the smallest unit of life that is classified as a living thing (except virus), and is often called the building block of life. Our cells regularly communicate with each other. They send and receive between 100,000 to 120,000 messages, known as bio-photons, per second. This speed of communication is superior to the velocity of light. If one cell does something different, then other cells know about it immediately. This was further discussed when Werner Meinhold discovered that cancer could be formed with Regressive Hypnotic Cellular Consciousness.

The cellular memory is the complete blueprint of our existence. Every lived moment is stored in our cellular memory. Our cells have complete information of us as a whole. Every cell is influenced by experiences we live even before the processes of prenatal stage or conception begin. The experiences undergone by a sperm and an ovum are stored in our cellular consciousness that can be readily accessed through hypno-Integrative therapy of depth psychology developed by Werner Meinhold. This technique also helps to integrate the malignant impregnations of past experiences through cellular consciousness and allows a person to experience a healthy, purposeful life.

Up until now we believed that the sperm penetrates the egg, which becomes the symbolic representation of the procreation process. Since we live in a world of duality, there is nothing that can be explained in a one-sided manner. In order for an initiator to exist there has to be a receptor, otherwise nothing is formed. When a sperm reaches an egg, the egg has to be available to receive it otherwise symbiosis cannot take place. The welcoming spiritual energy is the same as the arriving spiritual energy, and it is completely and beautifully balanced. Both sides help each other, both are equally important, co-existing and supporting each other such as Yin and Yang, Man and Woman. Only through this free-flowing exchange can gestation take place. Many of my clients have described a variety of experiences. Some explain in their experience as sperm-consciousness that they were chosen amongst many by the egg. These experiences confirm that the egg is not as passive as we imagine it to be. It has its own wisdom, own consciousness, own experiences and memories. This is why sometimes a sperm may fertilize an egg, or at other times the egg picks up the sperm and then the spirit enters to complete the process.

Upon writing this chapter, I have uncovered many more questions. Do all sperm feel the same as the one that was chosen? Did the special sperm feel differently than the others that caused it to be accepted by the egg? Does the egg know that it can only accept one sperm and has to let others die? What are the characteristics of an egg that receives more than one sperm? Is it possible for the egg to be willing to accept more than one sperm?

What happens in those cases where parents are trying for some time to get pregnant and have no success? I have not been able to answer many of these types of questions but one day I hope to. Or, perhaps one or more of you would be willing to share your experiences in order to shed more light on this subject.

One thing that I am sure of is the fact that there is a complete energetic and spiritual connection between an egg and a sperm. The same connection exists in our life and we connect with one another in almost each and every second of our life. It is a difficult notion to grasp and to accept by the intellect, but the same unconscious telepathic connection/communication has cured the most malignant of traumas and disorders during a holistic therapy session. I have borne witness to these miraculous moments not only in Canada but also in other parts of the world. Similar thing happens during fertilization where they help and support each other so that the natural process of conception can take place. The law of nature repeats in every form of life and is same everywhere.

The sperm is a single cell consciousness. Although the level of consciousness is somewhat muted, it is cognizant of its own awareness level, which is sufficient enough to do the task for which it was created. Yes, the spermatozoon has a consciousness. It has a consciousness of *Self*. It is aware that it exists, is alive and has a limited time span. It can feel and make a decision whether to continue its journey or to die there and then. He knows that he has to reach somewhere. He can feel the millions of other sperms running around him. He is conscious of the race where all of the spermatozoa are running for survival. He can even stop and sense that what he should do. He also carries the feelings of a possible future father. If the father had a fear then he carries that fear. Perhaps, at that time, the couple was not prepared to have a baby, or the baby could have been an unwanted child, or any other thought which might prevent the baby from taking birth. If the father felt happy and the couple had a strong desire to have a baby, then the sperm feels happy too and is warmly welcomed by an egg that can transform and transcend the gestation state into a positive and healthy birth of a baby.

Working with different clients, I have come across different and unique experiences. I remember one of my clients who felt the consciousness that her father had a strong desire to have a baby but mother did not because she wanted a separation. Her father had intentionally made his wife pregnant in order to remain with her. Although she had been a wanted baby by her father, she remained unwanted by her mother. She felt her mother's resistance towards her father, which consequently resulted in experiences as an adult where she had the same kind of resistance, anger and feelings of rejection towards the opposite sex. This is especially so in the case of men who wanted to be a part of her life.

A sperm not only has physical consciousness but spiritual consciousness as well. It is capable of feeling both good and bad. It appears to have strong feelings, and is "programmed" to know that it has a destination, which may or may not be reachable but that seems immaterial. What is critical to the sperm is to fully participate in the experience and fulfill its life's purpose.

> *"Experts believe this process may be nature's way of allowing only the healthiest sperm to fertilize the egg, thereby providing the best chances to produce a healthy baby."*

I do not agree with this statement. Every baby that is born is healthy and so is every unborn baby. Whether a baby is born with or without health problems, whether they took birth or were unable to complete their gestational life, each baby is always healthy. Although I always want every baby to be born healthy but judging them would mean not loving them. When we start seeing or receiving life as a whole, then everything starts making sense. We can choose to go beyond reason and simply "feel" life. We begin having an awareness of self, mindfulness of each other and of our surroundings while developing God-consciousness. We understand the purpose of our every action and everything that happens every moment of our lives. It is like putting all the pieces of a jigsaw puzzle together, and watching as the full picture clearly emerges and delivers its message to us.

Dr. Bruce Lipton's book *The Biology of Belief* sheds more light on cellular consciousness. According to his book, everything is part of a co-operative community of approximately fifty trillion single-celled citizens. Just as a nation is represented by the traits of its citizens, our human-ness is reflected in the basic nature of our cellular communities.

Although individual, each one has an evolved consciousness within which they share a mutual will for survival in the here and now (time) and in space. They work together to fulfill their daily functions within their state of self-consciousness. Even if one cell or group of cells is not ensuring its or communal survival, the other cells will have knowledge of that fact. According to Meinhold, when cells stop living their present wakefulness of "here and now" and go back in time to their archaic hypnotic stage, they begin producing the same group of cells we had since the creation of the Central Nervous System. This regression to their archaic consciousness of cells is today known as 'cancer.' If we draw them out of that archaic awareness to present-day wakefulness, then cancer can be disintegrated and those cells can resume their natural task and aim of ensuring mutual survival by living a harmonious and balanced life.

The base of all these cell behaviours resides in the information carried by the father and the mother. Can that DNA information be changed? In my experience, I have seen imbalanced cells transforming into healthy ones when the objective of the disease

28

is understood. Every disease is a path to health. The suffering is nothing but an opportunity to grow. If I remove your suffering, then that opportunity for growth for you is denied.

Every cell sings and shares a melody of life sending us messages through healthy or unhealthy body expressions. The solutions are created before the problems and the problems are a path to solutions. Problems help us grow. Self-awareness feeds the information to our cells and other body organs that are essential role-players that determine disease or wellbeing. The purpose of life becomes greater, broader, and different each time we move towards the next step of consciousness.

There is no fixed purpose of life and this often leads to confusion. If you do not ask the right question then you will never get the right answer. There are many books, marketing courses and Gurus peddling eternal happiness and promising to reveal to you your life's purpose.

A baby is formed with a mother cell and a father cell. The absence of either one of them will not result in the creation of a life. Perhaps, in the near future this might be possible, but in the present, there is no evidence or capability of human life being created without a father or a mother. This is the base of our life so it becomes the responsibility of each one of us to integrate this essence of duality in our daily life. Hence, the purpose of life becomes very simple as the life itself, and that is also the base of a healthy or unhealthy life. The simpler the life, the healthier we are and more likely to live.

The Purpose of Life

The purpose of life changes according to the consciousness we obtain. When submerged into sperm consciousness, our only purpose is to reach our destination and to unite. Likewise, the purpose of life changes almost every time we step into the next state of consciousness – an egg, gestation, foetus, baby, child, adolescent, adult and then old age. All these stages of life are fragmented into smaller yet different processes which begin and end no less than a fraction of every second.

Every new process is a new state of consciousness, and this is what determines the purpose of life for that very moment. For example, the purpose of life for a person who is dying would be to recover. The purpose of life may be for a single man would be to get married and have children; this can go on in multiple ways and directions.

So, you can see, the purpose of life cannot be determined or interpreted from a narrow worldly point of view. We live in a society, and therefore, our purpose is determined by society's rules and regulations. We cannot freely determine the purpose of life in the broader sense because it is so dynamic and changeable based on the shifting needs of the moment.

To figure out the purpose of life, we are willing to spend a great deal of money on costly courses delivered by professionals who simply regurgitate the information we already know. Or, they advance their own worldview of life based on social criteria, conditional reality and half-dualities, and expect us to find the elixir of happiness within them.

You cannot love others or yourself in parts. You cannot say that I love my right arm but I do not love my right leg. You could opt to say that but then it would definitely have dire consequences on your health, and that part of your body may go out of the balance and become unhealthy. Right questions create right answers. We cannot live a life based on narrow definitions. We cannot take an analytical approach in order to define or describe the quest we undertake to finding our life's purpose. Doing so would cause us to lose the joys and sorrows of living in the present moment; once gone, it is lost forever. Our cells store information that is genetically forwarded to our children and to the future generations. Only you have the power to change it. The choice is yours.

The Mystery of the "Special One"

Many of you may not agree with the idea of sperm consciousness and it may even create a great deal of controversy. Nevertheless, it is important for me to share this information as it can open the doors to new discoveries. I finished this chapter few months ago but recently, in my own practical experience I discovered that the sperm that fertilizes an egg is not a random one to successfully reach and fertilize the egg. In fact, there is only one sperm and it is the only one with just the right information and capacity to enter an egg and fertilize it. I will call it the "Special One" instead of the chosen one. The other sperms are naïve and merely move along as companions but do not possess the same capacity or the information to fertilize the egg. It means that their purpose is not to fertilize an egg but just be a part of the natural process of sperm-production.

There can be more than one sperm that could fertilize an egg, and when this occurs it usually results in twins or multiple births. Nevertheless, all sperms are aware of the presence of other sperms that carry the same information as them. They can also "feel" if the other special sperm would successfully reach the egg to result into a baby or not at all. This special one, with an awareness and capacity to fertilize the egg can perceive the presence of other similar sperms as well the ordinary ones. The special one is also guided in their journey by some force quite spectacular yet invisible. I do not have a name for it nor can I provide a concrete interpretation as it is beyond any sensorial perception.

From the above description we could say when it comes time to form a baby, the body creates that special sperm or sperms that will fertilize the egg and enable a new life to come into existence.

There is no such thing as the "chosen one" because all other sperms are just kind of cheerleaders and not really in the game. I perceive this to be a simultaneous pattern during conception, which I will call a *Triangulation Pattern* (i.e. Sperm and Egg join together and simultaneously a soul/spirit enters). The body, in its superior intelligence, creates the sperm, the egg awaits its arrival, the special sperm fertilizes the egg and the soul descends. There is a telepathic connection among all three. To be in a natural state of balance, harmony, and communication is the wisdom that resides within our bodies and it is beautifully revealed during the reproductive process.

This is the innate intelligence of our body at work, in harmony and in balance with nature; there are no coincidences, only causality. If there is any fear or trauma then the body does not initiate this pattern, and therefore it may take time to conceive or may result in not having the baby at all.

Now we know that the sense of telepathy works beyond time and limit. Does this mean that nature is intelligent enough to create a special sperm or sperms and save them for future fertilization in cases where sperm is donated or when artificial insemination is used?

If all of this is incorrect then it would be ridiculous to say that the soul descends every time there is a possibility of conception, or even during copulation, but if the sperm fails to reach the egg then the soul feels disappointed and returns to soul world to await the next opportunity to come back. Therefore, by implication, we must draw the conclusion that *all of the conditions for conception have to be perfectly lined up* so that the sperm-egg-soul triad could take place.

The Conscious Sperm

Although at this time my book has been published in India and many of the copies have already been sold, I still took the time to make it available in Canada, U.S.A. and in other parts of the world. Perhaps subconsciously I was waiting for my curiosity about sperm consciousness to be completely satisfied or maybe it was something else; whatever the case may be, at last, I am glad that I have received the complete answer to my questions regarding artificial insemination as this was previously left undiscovered.

My office happens to be in front of a centre where artificial insemination is done. Surprisingly, while working with some clients who underwent this process, my burning desire to find answers to my question became even more intense.

"If the special one is only created at the moment by the body when the time comes then what happens to cases where the sperm is donated or artificial insemination is used? And, if a large number of sperms is already out of the body then how can that special one come into existence to fertilize the egg?"

I am very pleased to share that I have discovered the answer to my questions, and I am ever so grateful to have come across those circumstances in which I was completely and logically able to comprehend the full birth process with sperm consciousness. I am sure that after reading about my discoveries, you will be equally amazed at how nature works its miracles with no margin for errors.

In order to answer this, first of all, I would like to change the name from "The Special One" to "The Conscious One." There can be more than one conscious sperm which may result in multiple births. The secret lies in the moment when the sperm gains consciousness with the arrival of the soul (or spirit) to take birth. This is the soul which transfers the consciousness to the sperm or sperms and waits for the sperm to reach an egg. This means that if the soul does not arrive to take birth then there will be no conception or pregnancy and this is why (besides other reasons described in this book) many parents cannot have a baby with natural methods or even with artificial insemination. What this implies is the fact that the presence of the soul is the first and most critical step in starting the pregnancy process. Does this mean that in order to have a baby we should not only be aware of the physical aspect but also the spiritual aspect of pregnancy? And, perhaps the spiritual aspect is far more important than a physical one?

It gives me goosebumps to write that my research leads me to believe that if it is the soul that dominates over the process from conception to birth, then the highly Conscious Soul could possibly bypass the natural process of the parents making love (which involves the essential process of father's sperm arrival to fertilize mother's ovum). Then, could this result in the birth of a highly ascended master whose purpose it is to guide humanity on the pathway to illumination and knowing the higher self?

Nothing makes sense and everything makes sense.
You decide.
Atul Mehra

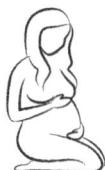

Chapter 4

The Eighteen Senses

Most of us are intrigued and puzzled when we hear about the eighteen senses. Would it surprise you to know that we use them consciously or unconsciously in our everyday lives? In order to understand and emerge from those hidden processes that control our lives, we must first acknowledge that these senses play a very important role in them. Understanding them has helped me to start living a more peaceful and balanced life. I am certain that this information will change your life one way or another.

We all know about the five physical senses. Rudolph Steiner explained additional seven senses in an effort to help us understand life in more depth. My life experiences as well as my clients have helped me to discover these natural yet hidden five basic senses. They are: the sense of Feeling, the sense of Awareness, the sense of Connection, the sense of Purpose, and the sense of Transformation. I attempt to describe their symbolism on a different level but the processes lived by the sperm are same as lived by any person during his whole life, which really makes it so interesting and provocative.

The Sense of Feeling

The word feeling has so many meanings that it becomes very difficult to justify its true significance. Feelings can be referred to as emotions or sensations experienced by the five senses, or to be in a particular state as a result of an emotion or a physical feeling. In fact, the sense of feeling cannot be described in words nor can it be rationalized. We can only experience in this state. When you feel yourself, you come to life. People create pain in order to feel alive.

Feeling is the first natural sense in all living things or with life. We do know that animals are able to recognize the difference between an enemy and a friend and react accordingly, i.e., with a fight or flight response or with mere curiosity. Pet owners may have witnessed this feeling in their pets.

Surprisingly enough, plants can feel too. The new research is in a field called plant neurobiology — which is something of a misnomer, because even scientists in the field don't argue that plants have neurons or brains. Michael Pollan, author of such books as *The Omnivore's Dilemma* and *The Botany of Desire* explains: "They have analogous structures. They have ways of taking all the sensory data they gather in their everyday lives ... integrate it and then behave in an appropriate way in response. And they do this without brains, which, in a way, is what's incredible about it, because we automatically assume you need a brain to process information." Pollan reasons that plants have the same senses as humans. In addition to hearing, taste, for example, they can sense gravity, the presence of water, or even feel that an obstruction is in the way of its roots, before coming in contact with it. Plant roots will shift direction, he says, to avoid obstacles. (http://www.pri.org/stories/2014-01-09/new-research-plant-intelligence-may-forever-change-how-you-think-about-plants).

We have to accept the fact that despite us knowing a lot about nature in general, this incredible information marks the beginning of new knowledge. Similarly, I am certain that new facts will come to light with respect to intrauterine life and pregnancy that will surprise us even more. I am sure that some of these I am already sharing with you.

The very first sensation of life felt by the sperm is with the sense of feeling. He feels himself and then comes into existence. The sense of feeling is the foundation of life. This feeling determines what we are going through in our life. If we feel good then we live peacefully; however, if we feel turmoil in our lives then we definitely need to learn the lessons in order to move towards a peaceful life. The feeling is the origin of our future actions. Sometimes people spend their whole lives to feel good, even risking their lives by breaking laws of nature. The sense of Feeling is a natural and automatic response to what is being lived at that very moment.

The sense of feeling is the most important sense for it is the basis of all other feelings; in other words, this is the first sense with which we are born. If I cannot feel myself then it means I am dead. The sperm feels itself, the egg feels itself and the soul feels itself, and in the period of gestation, the experience of threesome (i.e. Sperm, Egg and Spirit or Soul) is also the first experience that creates a complete human being. The sperm feels itself so it comes into existence and develops a sense of awareness of itself. His awareness helps him to develop a sense of connection with his surroundings and he finds his sense of purpose of being there is to "reach somewhere," and this becomes his sense of transformation. Each of the five basic senses goes through a continuous process that repeats from the beginning to the end of life. The same process is lived by the egg and the soul. Although this is a very "limited, small timespan process" lived by the sperm, it is nevertheless a complete process for the sperm cycle to finish.

The Sense of Awareness

Although the word awareness is considered to be the same as consciousness, I am of the opinion that there is a difference between the two. Awareness is having familiarity of a state or of something that exists in a particular moment. It could also be an understanding of a situation based on a feeling of that moment. Consciousness, on the other hand, is wakefulness or having an awareness of the totality of everything. Awareness can be small fragments of consciousness that lead us to experience a totality. Awareness is the second step of recognizing or perceiving "Self" for a sperm after feeling. The sense of awareness takes him to experience other senses, which are also parts of the sense of consciousness. In this regard, the conscious life can be the sum of all senses experienced leading to the constant state of being awake, thinking and knowing what is happening around you at all times. This leads to a continually expanding awareness of living here and now beyond the five physical senses. This is the experience of the sense of telepathy channeling toward consciousness. Experiencing these moments are higher meditation levels of the spiritual Self.

The Sense of Connection

The sense of Connection is one of most important senses. It is the state of being related to someone or something else. It brings us closer to someone or something. Being together or to be connected is also a part of loving someone or something. All of us would be isolated if we did not have this sense of Connection. The sense of Connection is also a form of communication. This communication can be between humans, human to animal, human to plants, human to non-living things or vice-versa. Nothing in the world would work without connection.

Everyone is in connection with everyone else; this is the whole point of creation. Regardless of whether you love or hate someone, the sense of connection is always present and working underneath.

How do you feel when you do not feel connected to someone but nevertheless you are connected somehow?

The sense of connection helps the sperm to link with his surroundings. His connectedness creates the cycle of action for which he has been created. Accepting help from his sense of connection, he increases his awareness of those moments to start an action. He is in a situation where he and his surrounding have the same origin and goal. He prepares himself for the cause so that he can fulfil his calling. What would happen if the sperm or one of us loses the sense of inner connection?

The Sense of Purpose
The sense of purpose is tied to action. The sperm identifies his purpose after connecting with his environment. Now he knows that he is destined somewhere and his journey has started. He starts moving with other millions of sperm, as this is what he has been programmed to do. Although he might be carrying the feelings of fear or happiness transferred by the father, he nevertheless continues to move towards his purpose against all odds.

The purpose of life is one of the most important senses the person looks for in his life. Most of us try to fill the emptiness based on our experiences in our mother's womb or during early childhood, and we confuse it with our purpose in life. The sense of purpose carries a very strong basic need of acceptance from others no matter what you do in life.

What exactly is the purpose of life? Is it to become an engineer, a doctor, a politician, an athlete, or a millionaire businessman? It can be anything but there is always a hidden desire to get recognition from others. You are likely to feel that in your life nothing fills you up, although you may have everything for which you yearn. There is always going to be something lacking sooner or later. Nothing is perfect and yet everything is perfect. The understanding of self or self-consciousness is the true purpose of life. Everything in life is nothing but experiences. You are the sum of your life's experiences. Your experiences and the surrounding environment create your purpose of life and all of your experiences serve their purpose. However, once you realize that purpose, it might create emptiness within you, and the question that arises is: "Now what?"

The sense of purpose guides us to ourselves, to our inner self. The moment we find ourselves, the quest stops and everything in life begins to make sense. Many things in our lives just do not make sense and that is because we are still not ready to understand them. The more you go far away or lose connection with your inner Self the more likely you are to experience hard lessons; nevertheless, that is a part of your holistic growth. There is a saying in India that sums up this experience succinctly: "The bird flies very high but it always comes back to his nest." You can fly far away from yourself but one day you have to come back to yourself to experience your purpose to recognize and accept who you really are.

The Sense of Transformation

Now speaking about the Sense of Transformation, I make reference to the experience when a sperm surrenders or transforms his life for a bigger physical and spiritual gain. This is known as gestation but in fact this is a celebration – a spiritual celebration of its own kind. He has transformed himself in something bigger. It is same as a caterpillar transforms into a butterfly. He does not know what will happen when he has reached his destination but he trusts the process. He trusts the information he carries with him and with the help of sense of life or transformation he completes his life cycle.

We are bound to time and space. The condition of here and now carries a basic understanding that when there is a beginning, there has to be an end as well. If we accept life then we have to accept death as well. Death is a continuation of life or transformation. The sense of transformation helps us to go through different experiences and stages. All emotions and relationships are pathways to understanding life. Life does not want to fight with us. It does not tell us to live sadly or happily. If I asked life, what should I do? I am sure life would say, "Just live." So live the way you want and live consciously. You have complete freedom and the choice between happiness and sadness. Cry when you love and feel happy when you share that love. The freedom to move freely in between two polarities is life.

Although we have come alone in this world, we live alone, and we must go alone, there is someone who always accompanies us from birth to transformation and that is the *self* or *I*. Learning to be with me first and in my own company is living my life.

These five basic senses work in every process of our lives. Just imagine if you feel sad because somebody has hurt you and when you connect with him or her, you begin a fight or engage in an argument. Now your purpose may be to make that person feel bad. In doing so, you are transforming or having a negative life experience. You can change your life easily if you start observing yourself using your basic senses. You will see all these five basic senses operate in every area of your life because you were formed on the basis of these senses.

The sense of touch
The baby starts connecting with the mother around 28 days from gestation and the first connection with the mother is through the Sense of touch. He is in need to feel his mother and at the same time he wants his mother to feel him. This assures his presence in the physical world. Meinhold claims, "being in mother's womb helps him to recognize that he is out of essence and now he is in existence and he can only feel that when mother feels it."

Although the receptors of touch are formed after 28 days of gestation, the process of touch happens much before this. That is the moment when the sperm and egg meet, and a spirit descends to form a baby. This is the contact with the mother. He is out of *nirvana* and in physical existence. He can only feel "into" existence if his mother also feels that way. The most important healthy development in this phase is "I feel that my mother feels me." Almost every client, upon entering this chronological stage of his life, feels happy when his/her mother declared that she is pregnant and it is at that precise moment that life starts. The sense of touch gives us the justification that we are accepted and recognized. Since ancient times, various cultural groups have held different ceremonies to celebrate a child's birth. While it is important to have a biological birth it is equally important to reaffirm the existence of the baby. This communication is required from the beginning.

The sense of touch is an internal sense of my limits and the beginning or connection of the world out of me. Touch is also a communication. The mother touches her stomach during pregnancy to caress the baby and he feels mother's love and acceptance and at the same time it transmits the sensations of pleasant calmness and meditation.

The sense of touch applies not only to the process of touching, but also to the feeling that something opposite to me exists and it verifies that I am in existence. All our senses work with the opposite. The absence of opposite is the absence of recognition. The presence of opposites or duality is lived throughout our lives. Have you ever considered how opposites create a balance in our life? They are not in competition with each other. They co-exist and co-create such events as day and night, life and death, youth and old age, good and bad, and so on.

The child confirms to the mother that she is pregnant and the mother confirms to the baby that he is in existence. This reciprocal balance creates the possibilities of a co-creation and co-existence. If the mother is afraid due to or anxious about her pregnancy, then the child will not feel accepted and he/she will spend a lifetime in a quest to feel accepted. Disorders such as bulimia, cutting his body or Attention Deficit Disorder (ADD/ADHD) develop within the person in an effort "to feel oneself." Whatever the form of the disorder, we have to uncover the hidden symbolism underneath it.

The Sense of Warmth

The sense of warmth contains a two-fold sense: 1) the physical experience of hot and cold temperatures and, 2) human or soul warmth or coldness. The sense of warmth is a very important sense that accompanies us in every moment of our lives. Everybody feels the physical sensation of hot and cold temperatures. But when it comes to human warmth, it goes beyond the physical into the deeper realms of the spirit. It is not only humans who are affected by the vibrations of warmth but so are plants and animals. There has been a great deal of research conducted on this and conclusions drawn about the presence of non-physical energy that moves between opposite poles.

The sense of warmth is connected with the sense of touch. A baby generally feels it around twelve days of intrauterine life. This is the second beginning after the contact. In a biological sense, when the mother's blood touches the baby's body for the first time, the sense of warmth develops. Blood is not only a thick, red liquid that we know, but also has a very deep spiritual significance such as the blood of Christ. It is the moment of union – yoga – of nesting in the mother's womb. The colour red also represents love and passion, so in other words, the sense of warmth can also be considered as a sense of love that is at the heart of creation. It is the unification of baby and mother. This is the mammalian consciousness that emerged out of the evolution of our central nervous system. This is the first time in evolutionary

43

history that love towards the child came into being. This sensation of warmth can only be felt when you are in your physical body. Heat is also a defense measure for fever. The high temperature experienced during fever is the only way that one can combat viral cells and destroy them.

In my experience, the sense of warmth starts much before the baby is formed. It is connected to the feeling of loving and being loved. This is the experience of acceptance. First, my mother recognizes me and then she accepts me (warmth). This warmth is the origin point for maintaining the sense of I (self). Having a sense of warmth provides me with the constant inspiration to live as an individual as well as in unison with others.

I have had clients who just could not feel the warmth or love of their mother. They were mostly those who were unwanted children or had issues in their childhood, and many describe their mother's behaviour towards them as cold. In those cases, the possibilities of having a pre-mature delivery were much higher than other cases. After going beneath the cold mask they could understand and connect the essential warmness of life. Some of them complained about cold legs or low blood circulation in their legs.

Again, the question remains: what exactly is the sense of warmth? In my experience the sense of warmth starts even before the baby is formed. Feeling warmth is the state or sensation of being warm. The radiating warmth of the sun, the genuine warmth of a smile, a tender warm heart, a hearty warm welcome and a big, warm hug trigger a set of emotions where we feel good and accepted. The word warmth can trigger so many sentiments including friendliness, amiability, geniality, cordiality, kindness and so on. All these sensations can be lived and experienced with a mere mention of the word warm. Can warmth be a synonym for love?

The sense of warmth starts exerting influence even before the baby is conceived. There are different situations and scenarios with respect to this, but in this case we will assume that the biological parents will take care of their son or daughter. Taking that into account, it is important for them to feel a sense of warmth and love between them. According to the general rule, if mom and dad deeply love each other, then the baby will be formed with complete warmth and love. If parents have doubt, fears or feel that getting pregnant was a mistake, then this information is transmitted and it creates possibilities for a cold welcome into the world for the baby. My recommendation based on my experience would be for parents to work with the definition of the word *warmth* in their lives and for those do not feel warmth during pregnancy.

The Sense of Balance

The sense of balance is one of the important senses in life. We need balance in everything. All things are in balance and we have to maintain that balance between the polarities. Everything that moves has a fixed, center point (also known as an axis). Although that fixed point does not move, it serves as a point of reference. If I cannot feel my center then I do not have a reference point and I will have difficulties in receiving and interpreting the world.

Have you ever wondered what is the center of our body? Majority of people would point at their belly button; however, if you were to use a measuring tape then you would find that it is more or less located at our genitals. In Indian traditional meditation techniques, it is referred to as the *root chakra* and it connects us with mother Earth. There are many other symbolisms connected with that area of our body. The center of our body also refers to our existence and it is connected with a sense of balance.

The sense of balance is developed in a baby every time the mother moves or walks. The sense of balance helps us to find our center and that has to be found inside us. If my center is not in me then it means it is out of me. So someone or something else has to fill that emptiness in order for me to feel complete. The small, peaceful movements during childhood can create a sense of balance but strong movements can lead to sense of imbalance or possibly traumas later in life. I have worked with many clients who feel deep anxiety as adults because their mother fell down, had an accident, or suffered physical abuse at the hands of her husband at the time of her pregnancy.

We need to recognize the importance of balance in intrauterine development. We need to feel that the beginning of our center is the navel but changes later when our legs grow, symbolizing freedom, and the center changes to the location of the genitals. In utero, the baby communicates with its mother through the umbilical cord connected at the navel, but then the communication in adult life changes into sexuality. Many communications, however, are not only sexual intercourse. After birth the child is rocked in a cradle, which becomes a substitute for the womb and continues to develop a sense of balance within the child.

Everything in our universe is in a state of balance. Everything supports the other in order to create a natural balance. Everything from the inhalations and exhalations of our breath to the planets are maintaining that balance. In life, we do not feel pure happiness or sadness, but rather combination of both. We need to find our own balance from our experiences. When we feel pain, we cry or feel hurt but we do not stay in pain for the rest of our lives. Sometime after, we feel happiness again and when we are happy, we laugh. This is what makes us human. Finding that balance between two opposing polarities is essential: I wish to fly like a bird but fear causes me not to jump from the roof of a building, and so I still live. Later, I am so inspired by my wish to fly like a bird that I gather my courage and creativity to construct an airplane so I could fly in the sky. Thus, growth comes from extremities and not from center.

Balance is necessary in each and every moment of our life. Therefore, pregnant women are highly recommended to integrate movement into their daily routine. Walking, yoga, prenatal exercises under the supervision of a healthcare professional are all very useful for a baby to develop the sense of balance.

The Sense of Hearing

The sense of hearing is also connected with the sense of balance. Although in the evolution of the central nervous system, the sense of hearing is much older than the sense of sight, it is considered to be the most important sense for humans. Hearing allows us to communicate with each other by receiving sounds and interpreting speech. The baby listens to mom and dad conversations and other sounds to identify and interpret whether he is loved or rejected.

Imagine if we are engaged in an activity and somebody comes up behind us and shouts – would you be startled or even scared to death? When watching a horror movie, those sounds scare us and since our unconscious mind cannot differentiate between reality and imagination, we are prone to feel negative effects on our subconscious mind. Likewise when we listen to gentle, peaceful sounds we feel a sense of tranquillity and calmness. We can think, react and take correct decisions when we have relaxed mind and peaceful thoughts. Decisions based on violent, impulsive and coerced situations generally tend to have negative outcomes. Don't you agree?

Baby feels acceptance or rejection through sounds. Strong, violent sounds scare him and peaceful loving sounds make him feel accepted. They work directly on his self-esteem, confidence and his future adult behavior. Sometimes I wonder how they would affect those babies who witness violent scenes in movies or they are acting in the movies. Being exposed to such an environment would surely affect their lives in some way later on.

The sense of hearing has a very important role in creating a connection between the baby and the parents, or with others around. Since baby cannot see his parents, all of them could feel a sensation of being loved or rejected after identifying the sounds they hear. They felt peaceful moments and went to sleep when they heard their mom singing; but they felt stressed when exposed to scary, violent, and strong sounds.

Baby listens to everything and absorbs it for future development. One of the biggest recommendations I can make is to avoid arguments during pregnancy and even after when the baby is born. During a session, one of my clients remembered how his parents used to yell at each other and generally had a very violent relationship between them. He suffered a great deal in his mother's womb, which caused deafness in his life. The symbolism of ears is to listen and when I cannot avoid listening to hateful and scary sounds, it can trigger deafness. Violent and noisy arguments have also been one of the causes of premature delivery in some cases.

In biology, the sense of hearing is also connected with the sense of balance. From a holistic point of view it is not only a physical balance but also a spiritual balance. Loss of balance is also one of the symptoms of vertigo.

It would be valuable to play melodious symphonies of various classical musicians or talented artists to help the baby stimulate his development in a positive way. You can always consult your doctor or a healthcare professional working in this field. I hope they recognize how important positive sounds are to a developing baby. Heartbeat is a rhythm that can be found in different kinds of music, the stronger it is, the more interesting it becomes.

Mothers-to-be who perceive the idea of a baby growing inside them may want to start talking to him or her, and encourage the father to do the same. It will not be all in vain because the baby can hear you and feel deeply connected to you through your voice.

Medical research claims that the hearing in babies develops around the sixth week of pregnancy, which is true from a scientific standpoint. However, the spirit can also "hear" and therefore you ought to begin talking to your baby the moment you perceive that you are pregnant. Your conversation about or with the baby can create an impression on its developing psyche. The voices, tones, and sounds he or she hears and experiences are the gateway to the birth environment. The soft, melodious, and loving sounds create good positive experiences but constant harsh, angry, and loud noises can create sensations of fear, anxiety, or rejection. Apart from pregnancy, even in everyday life, noisy and intense arguments are not good for your children's mental health.

The Sense of Movement

The sense of movement is one of the senses of self-identity and has a direct connection to the sense of self or I. Movement is connected to life and is the direct opposite of death. This is one of those critical senses that sets us apart from plants.

An unborn baby starts to physically move by about 10 weeks of pregnancy but he still carries the consciousness of movement from the spermatozoon. The legs and the arms are connected with the sense of movement and possess their own sensors. In fact, the sense of movement parallels the sense of freedom. Our consciousness plays a very significant role in order to understand the sense of movement and its relation to the sense of freedom. Animals have less consciousness than human beings. An animal moves when he chases its prey. It is just following its instincts but that is not freedom. It is simply the stimulation of a reflex that causes the movement. The space I can occupy is the commencement of the sense of freedom.

The diseases connected with the sense of movement can be paralysis of the legs and arms. I cannot move because I am fixed or the conditions in my life do not allow me to move; or it maybe that my parents control me excessively and I do not have my own space and freedom. Many of my patients recall their memories of having limited space in their mother's womb, which later manifested as having less freedom, or pleasing others, or just finding ways to escape from the responsibilities of life. Once they understood these unconscious processes, they were able to emerge out of this state.

My recommendation for the mother would be to devote some time on simple physical activities such as walking or stretching whenever possible. This will help the mother feel well, and of course, if mother feels good then baby feels good too.

The Sense of Smell

The power of smell originated in our primitive state. A male bear can smell a female bear in heat from a distance. Sometimes I wonder if a primitive man had the same capacity to detect the mating desire of a primitive woman. Could it be that she emitted some sort of a scent from her body, causing a male to be sexually attracted to her? Have we lost this natural ability because of our exposure to and desire for artificial perfumes and scents? If so, then can the pheromones used in perfumes help to attract a man towards a woman?

Generally speaking, a majority of the senses we utilize are done in an effort to experience closeness with ourselves. For instance, in using the sense of movement, I move to be always near me; in using the sense of hearing, the closer I hear, the better it is. The sense of smell has the ability to perceive distant signals. It is our first response to stimuli. We can smell food before we can taste it, or we smell something burning even though we cannot see the flames. Most animals connected to earth have an incredible sense of smell. One of the best examples of this is a dog whose olfactory system is far more advanced than that of humans'. This is why dogs are used to detect explosives, illegal drugs and currency, items from missing persons, blood, and even contraband electronics. According to the ancient Indian chakra (energy centres) system, one of the characteristics of the element earth is smell. In ancient Egypt, when people suffered from flatulence, they were made to smell anise essence so that their intestinal gases would be expelled through the anus or the root chakra.

If I change something in my own smell then it means that there is a change in me. Almost every pregnant woman notices a change in her sense of smell during pregnancy, which is an early sign of pregnancy. Smell plays a strong role in emotional connection and in the bond between a mother and her baby. The mother's smell during pregnancy helps the baby feel secure and safe with her because his primary connection with the mother after birth is through the senses of smell, touch, and voice. The memories connected with smell during pregnancy helps him to continue his experience in his mother's presence; for example, the amniotic fluid in which the baby breathes and floats while in the womb further helps to attract the scent of breast milk after birth.

Smells can affect the baby during pregnancy. Prolonged use of good or bad smells during one's pregnancy can cause the baby to be naturally attracted towards those smells more than the other ones. I have always wondered if our smell is somehow responsible for creating an attraction between two people of the opposite sex – even unknown to them – and for having a baby together.

Different that the other senses, the sense of smell operates with the olfactory system, which is a direct part of the brain. It does not need a nerve to the brain like other senses. Light is a form of energy we receive through our eyes, and this energy converts into a binary system, which is indirect: light or no light.

Meinhold states that the molecule of smell is directly connected to the brain. It is like being in communion with the brain. When I sense the smell of a woman or a partner, whether consciously or unconsciously, then I recognize this smell as my partner and I communicate and create a communion with this person. If I cannot smell you, I cannot recognize you. In our consumerist world, we have a plethora of scents and perfumes available to us, so we do not accept each other as naturally as we used to. We need to put on a mask in order to accept others.

The Sense of Life

Rudolf Steiner explained the sense of life about being well and living in harmony. Meinhold explains it further by taking it into a deeper level – all vital body processes are connected and have to have a centre for this condition to work, In this case, the mother becomes the center for all these vital processes.

He further explains how cells, if not working in harmony, can destroy life and create malignant diseases. These processes he calls a sense of life or vegetative. He also emphasizes the importance of abstaining from smoking or drinking because these are alien substances to the body that could destroy the harmony of cells and other vital processes.

The sense of life is one of the most important senses. If I am not me then I am someone else. I will allow other strange energies to occupy that space. The word life can be described as existence, a way of life or opposite of death. My existence is based on the space I occupy because without me there would be emptiness. The baby occupies that space in his mother's womb, which gives mother the indication that she is pregnant. Although he is a different human being, his condition is one with the mother. He is in symbiosis with the mother. The mother is opposite to him so that he can recognize his existence. He connects with the mother and through the mother's experiences, feelings and thoughts; he creates his sense of life

Many parts are repressed in our unconscious and we need to make the unconscious conscious. This requires a lot of work and effort because we can never have complete knowledge of the Self. The harmony of vital life processes can only be possible if we are in harmony with ourselves. From our origins we are all healthy, but biologically, if we happen to live a life with shortfalls and health challenges then we must accept them.

If we are not in our body psychically then life will come to an end because there is no development. What remains after death is the spiritual self. The "self" of now is part of the spiritual self but it needs a body. The body is not something we have but something we are. If we do not treat our body with respect and love then we are not treating our higher level with respect. The body needs much more acceptance.

Meinhold emphasizes the importance of cellular awareness in the mother's womb. It is important for every cell that wants to duplicate to know if it matches the needs of his environment around him. Too many duplicate cells generate problems and all vital processes of the cells must be in harmony with each other. The genes of the cell have a task to ensure that duplication process is being done correctly. When strong radiation, toxic defenses, or psychic wounds damage a gene, it cannot properly control the other cells. When mutation takes place cells need to be repaired but if it gets out of hand then the gene has the task of destroying the cells. These cells cannot be consciously accessed because the entire process takes place as if it were a concert.

If I am not complete within me then something else from outside has to occupy that space in me. We have to occupy by ourselves. For example, if I smoke or take drugs, then these are alien substances that occupy that emptiness. They are strange external energies that cause self-destruction. They do not contain the possibility of creating communication between cells. The harmony of vital processes can only be harmonic if we are in harmony with ourselves. The task is to live a happy, joyful life.

We need to recognize healthy ways of living because, in a biological sense, we are all healthy, and if we live a life with a shortfall then we must accept it.

Not only do pregnant women need to avoid these alien substances in life but also everyone else. Finding solutions for our physical and mental shortfalls and living in harmony within us and around us is what characterizes the sense of life.

The Sense of Taste

The baby's sense of taste starts to develop early in pregnancy and he cultivates special tastes and has preferences for foods consumed by the mother during her pregnancy, even years later or sometimes for the rest of their life. This is why it is very important for the mother not to smoke, drink alcohol or use other illegal drugs during pregnancy. The baby can have serious developmental problems as a result of any of these harmful substances. Do drug-consuming mothers give birth to babies who are prone to drug addiction in the future?

During the first two months of pregnancy, the taste buds start forming and these receptors begin to recognize various tastes such as sweet, salty, or bitter. The baby in utero can suck his thumb from the 20th week onwards and this helps to grow those taste bud receptors. Sucking thumb is also a natural symbol for sucking mother's nipple or breast-feeding in the near future. From my clinical experience, I always recommend breast-feeding after the baby's birth because breast milk provides protection from diseases, and also helps to create a bond with the mother. I recognize that there may be circumstances where breast-feeding is not possible. It is healthier for a mother to talk to the baby to explain that she would love to breast-feed but this is not possible and she loves him no matter what, rather than feeling guilty about it later on. I also recommend giving complete attention to the baby during breast-feeding instead of being engaged in some other activity.

Many of my patients have interpreted this distraction as a form of rejection from the mother, which later adversely affected their adult life.

Symbolically, taste is a part of sympathy and antipathy not only with food but also with smell. Taste buds should be developed from early childhood so that the feeding does not become any kind of training. Exposing the baby to a variety of flavors can achieve this. In thinking about the taste of food, we must include the taste of a kiss. I know someone who never kissed his children in their early childhood when he smoked cigarettes or drank alcohol; but later he completely overcame these addictions because his children asked him to quit. Sympathy and antipathy are very important to develop in childhood. The life of a baby pre and post-pregnancy until the cutting of the two front teeth is a life of reflection from the information received from the mother and the outer world is a reference to know himself.

The Sense of Telepathy and/or Thought

"Telepathy" is derived from the Greek terms "*tele*" meaning "distant" and "*pathe*" meaning "occurrence" or "feeling". So it is the distant communication between people of thoughts, ideas, feelings, sensations and mental images, etc., involving mechanisms that cannot be understood in terms of known scientific laws. It is also known as thought transference. So, in simple words, telepathy is the communication between two minds, separated over a distance without using any of our known sensory channels or physical interaction.

At some point in our life, we all have experienced telepathy. You may be thinking of a person, and you receive a call from that person, or when you say something before another person and he says, "Oh, I was going to say the exact same thing!" In my life I have felt it more than often especially with the people I love. Even while doing an activity, I receive mental images that are astonishing.

Sigmund Freud termed telepathy as a regressive, primitive faculty that was lost in the course of evolution, but which still had the ability to manifest itself under certain conditions. Psychiatrist Carl G. Jung thought it more important. He considered it a function of synchronicity. Psychologist and philosopher William James was very enthusiastic towards telepathy and encouraged that more research be put into it. (http://www.themystica.com/mystica/articles/t/telepathy.html)

Based on the research done by Werner Meinhold, the sense of telepathy and the sense of thought are combined. According to him, this is a very special sense as only human beings can think. What we learn in school is not thinking because most of what is being studied by school children is based on repeating what others have already thought. All of us have to think, as thinking is the only pathway to original ideas and creativity. In school we learn to ruminate and regurgitate, but we do not learn how to communicate. Think how to think and not to repeat.

Thought can also be considered to be a part of the sense of Telepathy. What I think and feel is also a form of communication that is telepathic. The deepest levels within us are original and enter into direct communication. In direct communication there are no means of communication, nerves or senses but rather, there is a direct participation on a higher level where all of us contribute a part of our being. The sense of thought when it becomes telepathic does not need time. If you become rays of sunlight then you need time. Direct communication does not need time and space between the transmitter and the receiver. We do not know who sends and who receives the message but it is by mutual consent and they produce mutual information simultaneously and instanteously.

Baby connects with mother through a telepathic connection. What mother feels or lives during pregnancy become the first lessons in a baby's life and later in life he tries to live unconsciously through those experiences. If a mother feels bad, depressed or anxious, then these sentiments of rejection or acceptance are transferred into the child via this telepathic connection. I will discuss this later in the chapter entitled, "Mother and Baby Communication."

Telepathy has also been used to connect with dead people because they live outside of space and time. It is not recommended because we do not know what is on the other side and may lead to dangerous experiences.

We need to reach out with love and peace to the dead. Accept the death of a loved one with love and grace. God forbid but should a child die while in the womb, it is safe to say that he has lived a complete life. No feelings of guilt or sadness will help but only love will heal. The loved one who has died has to continue his spiritual journey, and while it is difficult to accept, I do not recommend that we retain a hold on him/her for our own needs. Many of my clients who had lost their babies during pregnancy were holding sentiments of guilt and fear, and were afraid of losing another child again in a future pregnancy. The sense of telepathy helped them to understand that it was not their fault and also the fact that it was not the right time for that baby to be born. This understanding alleviated the burden they had been holding for so long, resulting in a better and more contented life. If a baby dies in the mother's womb then it is difficult for the mother to let the pain go away because the only connection with the baby is now through the pain of loss. If she loses her pain then she loses her baby or that connection with the baby too. It requires a great deal of effort to process these feelings of guilt. Even though other methods work very well, the pain still remains trapped in those memories. The sense of telepathy has helped these mothers to find the malignant connections and release them, allowing them to live in the present.

In many ways it is very difficult to talk about cause and effect. Where does cause begin and where does effect begin? We live in a world where we cannot control certain situations. A minimum movement of a system can change everything and fortunately this change can occur on the spiritual level. The telepathic sense is a direct communication link, which connects with and understands the tasks and experiences connected to our *karma*. If we can arrive at this understanding, then in this system there is no such thing as "guilt."

We need to work on ourselves so that we can free ourselves from the malignant telepathic connections that control us daily at an unconscious level, thus creating pathways to dissatisfaction and negativity. We need to explore and understand what is hiding underneath these malignant energies and what factors are causing them. Apparently, the receptor organ of the body for the sense of telepathy is the pineal gland, which is, according to recent studies, being adversely affected by the use of cellular phones.

The advancement of new technologies, such as the Internet and mobile phones, play an important role in weakening social ties because they create a geographically diverse communication network and pull people away from traditional social settings, neighbourhoods, organizations, and public spaces that have traditionally forged strong community networks and connections. Ironically, we use tools of communication but we are communicating less and becoming more socially isolated. This form of communication is based on an imbalance of power. Power that is not expressed transforms into violence against us or against others.

Karma is "action" or "doing". Working with our sense of telepathy, we can better understand our connection with the dead and death. It can even help us understand on a deeper level that it is not very important to speak about the World War but to decisively act in order to prevent or put a stop to current wars and conflicts. If we do not recognize the significance that history holds for our present and our future, then we have learned nothing. Our integral consciousness has a lot to do with it. An individual soul communicates a message to us, and so does the soul of a city. We are all interconnected and have a telepathic connection to each other; we were created to live in telepathic harmony and not be separate from others.

The Sense of Sight

Eyes play a very important role in our life. It gives us the sense of sight. Approximately 70% of our daily activities depend upon our sense of sight. Our eyes allow us to see and interpret the interaction between light and darkness. Can you imagine your life without sight or without the use of your eyes?

"Eyes are the windows to our soul" is a popular expression. When we look into someone's eyes we may be able to see pain, anger, or some other emotion. How confident we feel when we talk to someone while looking into each other's eyes. Even the process of falling in love starts with an eye contact. The transmission rate of the ear nerves is faster than the eye. It may also be that the image information is larger and therefore takes longer to reach the brain.

We live in the here and now (time and space), but when we become aware of both, they cease to exist. We could never perceive here and now if we depended on our physical senses.

The distance travelled by light waves is faster than sound waves, but if we are closer to the source of sound then it appears as faster. We are under an illusion about the here and now because our brain makes it seem so; in fact, the signals reach the brain at different times and at different wave velocity but the brain converts them into the same speed the moment they arrive. The moment we sense or receive the description of reality, it is no longer there. These senses are not very precise or reliable tools. We also have our filters to see what we see. Everybody will describe a scene differently based on what he sees. A good example is when different people watch a movie and describe it very differently to another person. Developing a sense of telepathy eliminates the need for processing of senses and also removes the time-space barrier.

I can recognize a person through his/her eyes. Meinhold says, "When a baby is born through natural birth, he comes out and looks for his mother's eyes. How does he know that he has to find her eyes if the baby is born with reduced vision? My impression is that he recognizes that he is at the right place with the right person." The sense of sight is a very important sense in the development of freedom together with the sense of movement. Sight cannot only sense light but also sense shadow.

The Sense of Word with Speech Sense

Speech is symbolic of us evolving as human beings. The day we started talking or developed the sense of speech we became human beings, and this marks a major difference between animals and us. We developed the capacity to identify the functional meaning of the word as well as to think and to respond. When we can think in words, we can fathom the deep mysteries of the universe through the depths of philosophy or soar with the wings of mysticism. The sense of word starts from intrauterine life and this is the connection with the mother. It grows and develops to the first four years of life, after which the child separates from the mother and starts to use a more sophisticated form of speech.

The use of soft and accepting unconditional loving words in intrauterine life plays a very healthy and important role in baby's formation and his future life. This sense is also connected with the sounds and tones perceived by the baby. Baby dislikes the loud arguments between his parents but repeated exposure cause him to learn how to argue which will set him up for a dysfunctional life in the future. It is beneficial for a mother to avoid watching horror or violent movies with fearful and scary sounds. Likewise, music containing strong beats, inappropriate lyrics, and loud noises can create different unhealthy learning patterns.

The Sense of Self or I

The sense of self or I is connected to recognizing the real meaning behind that word. Every human being is an individual and each individual is different. He interprets the self according to his own personality.

The baby enters into intrauterine life like a clean, new computer that has no program written into it as yet. His parents and other significant people may impose certain conditions upon his birth (e.g., preferences such as giving birth to a boy rather than a girl, blue eyes, blonde, to become a singer as an adult, etc.) during his intrauterine life, forcing him to adopt a mask that separates him from his real self and takes him away from his true purpose.

He assumes someone else's characteristics in order to gain familial and social acceptance, so that his existence could be validated and approval would make him feel worthy. This causes the symbiotic deficit and also prohibits the natural and healthy development through early childhood stages. It later finds its balance in physical or mental diseases. The mother imposes an unconscious condition in her baby's intrauterine life, generating a deficit in the child that corresponds to that life period which is now prohibited to develop, and later the same is then connected with the conditional acceptance imposed on the couple.

This condition of acceptance to the other is part of the drama of life. While it is true that the mask allows one to interrelate and feel accepted first by the mother and later by society, the fact remains that it ends up limiting the person because he confuses this mask with his true self. This prevents other childhood phases from developing in a healthy way. The idea of first "to have" then "to be" is transmitted in the intrauterine life. If similar events occur again, the person finds himself filling that emptiness for rest of his life. For example, if I have a car, a house, a family, and a steady job, etc. then others accept me and I have earned a right to live. If any one of the above is missing then I do not exist, I am worthless, and I do not have a right to live. There can be many different similar unconscious patterns depending upon the life person in living, and if they are explored and understood through certain meditation techniques then a person can live a free and contented life. We are our own mirrors and in our reflection we must have the ability to recognize that whether we are centred or not.

We can only recognize our present situation at this very moment. If we imagine that situation then we come away from the present. It means living a life in the "here and now": when I eat, I only eat and do not read or talk because food deserves its own acceptance. When I sleep then I only sleep and do not think about what I am going to do tomorrow. I am completely present with that activity at that very moment and nothing else occupies me. The self is important for all these experiences, and we need to validate ourselves through everything we learn.

Meinhold says, "The self or I has different levels; he is a baby in womb, a child, an adult and also the future life he would live. The self is about the consciousness of his whole life, his spiritual being and as an individual and we do not have to find it in the brain." The self is not only about the consciousness of the existence but also the consciousness of himself. The only security we have is the consciousness of our spiritual self, which we are born with, and we cannot seek refuge in another person, money or anything else. This self is also the need to know the other self. If I cannot develop myself then I cannot recognize the other self. We have possibilities of expanding and developing our consciousness, our love and our freedom.

The Sense of Perception

Although I had previously thought of including the sense of perception in my book, I felt some sort of a resistance in the form of confusion when explaining the basic five senses as experienced by the sperm in a mother's womb. So I gave myself some time to reach a deeper understanding about this through meditation and working with my clients. I finally decided to include it here as the 18th sense. I realized that the sense of perception could not be ignored as it intimately connects to all of the senses and therefore plays a very important role in our daily lives. I thought it would be very similar to the sense of awareness, and indeed I did later discover that the sense of perception has a direct connection with the sense of awareness. The more you perceive, the more aware you become and the more aware you become, the more you can perceive. This is incredible, isn't it?

The word perception is derived from the Latin word *percipere* (seize, understand) to *"perceptio"* meaning, "perceive" or "perception." According to the Merriam-Webster dictionary, the simple definition of perception is 'the way you think about or understand someone or something." This definition is fine to understand in general terms but it does not fit into our context of intrauterine life because we know that a baby cannot think or understand while in its mother's womb. This treasured dictionary further explains perception as a fuller definition in these words: "awareness of the elements of environment through physical sensations". This definition is much closer to what I want to explain. The perception is a small moment before awareness. The baby can feel physical sensations. He feels and perceives mother's emotions and thoughts and then adds them to his limited yet complete awareness of that moment, later using it as a base of his future experiences. That moment of perception is a very delicate moment and it has a direct impact on our daily life. If the base of our perception has been connected with the awareness of negative events and experiences, then that person will resist living and understanding positive situations and experiences. He will have a general negative attitude towards life and although maybe, everything is positive and smooth, he would still have doubts and desolation inside and he would feel incomplete in his everyday life. Do you know someone who lives by those standards?

The sense of perception basically connects with all senses. The sense of perception helps us understand all other senses. If we fail to develop any one of our senses, then we cannot have the "perception" of what that particular sense provides us with and we lose that information for the rest of our life.

Now many of us can get a little bit entangled between the two words "intuition" and the sense of perception. Interestingly, perception is also a moment before intuition and it is different from intuition. The word "intuition" comes from the Latin verb *intueri* translated as "consider" or from late Middle English word intuit, "to contemplate." Intuition is a hunch, an idea or a guess independent of any reasoning process. It may manifest itself as a quick insight or an immediate apprehension but it is a onetime event. Now you cannot live a continuous intuitive life. It happens once in a very particular moment and stops and it may occur later but we don't know when. On the other hand the sense of perception is a continuous process. It is working 24/7. We perceive things based on our experiences and we take decision based on that too. It means the sense of perception plays a very important role to what we call "success" according to the materialist point of view of our life. Surprisingly, intuition can fail but the sense of perception cannot. What do you think?

You might have heard a sentence "How did you know I would drop by?" "Oh, I don't know. It must have been intuition." Unfortunately, this is not intuition but rather is the sense of telepathy; nevertheless the sense of perception plays an important role with the sense of Awareness.

Now we can fully appreciate how important the sense of perception is in our lives; it accompanies us even before birth and through every moment in our lives. One example might be this: you are walking home alone in darkness and suddenly you feel goose bumps all over your arm and neck; at that time your sense of perception is active, alerting you of the fact that something is wrong… Boo.

The sense of perception is recognition and interpretation of sensory information. It can also be our response to that information perceived. We perceive and judge the information and then we interact with our surroundings. Our previous experiences also play an important role as they allow or deny the received information. For example, if someone has lied to you a few times, you might entertain his talk with disbelief but maybe this one time he says something in a way and you perceive that he is telling you the truth. That is the sensory information you perceived, interpreted and decided to help him this time in spite of all those previous experiences.

The sense of perception is a very important process in our daily lives, and helps us live a more balanced and conscious life. I think it can be beneficial for every one of us to consider and use these 18 senses in our everyday life. It really makes sense.

Unconditional love cannot be lived without
understanding the conditions.
Atul Mehra

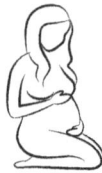

Chapter 5

Unconditional Love

Love is an emotion that binds us to others and to ourselves. It is present every single moment in our lives. It has many faces: affection, attachment, kindness, compassion, benevolence, sympathy, understanding, friendliness, care and so on. It can be any idea or a feeling that gives us a sensation of connectedness to others. Even the purpose of creation is Love.

The notion of love as an emotion must also include its counterpart, hate. This is the absence of love, badly expressed love or inaccessible love. Although negative, hate is present in all of us and simultaneously binds us to others but with one main difference: there is either a marked lack of understanding or a lack of human kindness, or both. Love, on the other hand, is an energy that connects us to every living and non-living thing. God forbid, when we lose a loved who has been a part of our life for some time, we miss them a great deal. In fact, love in perpetuity remains a mysterious and extraordinary emotion for mankind, and there is still a great deal to comprehend about it.

Love as consciousness is beyond duality. It is a critical part of our daily lives that demands our understanding from a holistic point of view. The word holistic is derived from the Greek word "*holos*" meaning all, whole, total or entire. We cannot separate ourselves from us. What this means is that I cannot love you or myself in parts. Furthermore, I cannot say that I love my eyes but not my nose, or, that I love your arms but I hate your face. In order to love, you have to accept the whole person. Since we are all connected to one another, we need to learn to accept ourselves as we all are. If you accept others with many conditions attached, then you also accept yourself with conditions many more than that. Start accepting yourself as you are and you will start accepting others as they are. The more you accept yourself, the more you accept others and vice versa.

This statement is equally effective for the baby who comes to share his life with you. He is the soul who is attracted to you for the love you have or will have for him. He has decided to share his entire life with you and to be with you to share the good and bad moments of life. And the same goes for you and your attraction to him. You also decided to be a part of his life. This whole process is reciprocal and mutual. There is no binding contract between both of you, nor does either one of you need to seek the other's approval to enter it. It is a completely natural process. It happens to everyone, no matter what family you belong to or in which part of the world you took birth and grew up. The loving arrival of the baby from its mother's womb is the same in any part of the world.

A very dear friend and mentor asked me the other day about the different challenges I face when I treat my clients with different backgrounds. He was amazed when I responded that while working with many clients of diverse cultural, linguistic, and national backgrounds in Canada, I observed that all of them suffered more or less from the same problems during their childhood. So, I faced absolutely no challenges with their treatment, as the solutions are universal for all human beings. All of them lived in-between polarity. This means that they either lacked love or had excess of love or something in-between. This is what makes me feel so excited about the fact that even though we are all different, we are all born as humans and so, all our problems are also human; similarly, our solutions have to be human solutions. Although it sounds funny, it is an honest experience that I have had my entire life. It is the same for doctors and surgeons. The diagnosis and the treatment are identical for same diseases for all the people in different parts of the world.

From there we can start understanding the basis of unconditional love. Like the medicine that goes inside our bodies, love acts in a similar way against diseases without thinking and differentiating between people. Love heals all in the same way, regardless of one's nationality, cultural or linguistic backgrounds. Irrespective of where you may be, you need to feel the same unconditional love for your baby. I am not telling you to be perfect because nobody is, but you can always try your best to avoid opinions, advice, and situations that could force your baby to feel conditioned. Perhaps, you have had a heated argument with your husband on any topic or something else. Your emotions make you feel out of control, or perhaps you become nervous, angry or fearful. Remember, your baby absorbs these emotions. Whatever a mother feels, whether or not it is connected with the baby itself, it is transferred to the unborn that is compelled to feel concerned about its mother's feelings and carries it for the rest of its life. If you experience any of these situations while pregnant, the first and most important thing is to become aware that you have lost your balance and it may affect your baby. Calm down and talk to your baby to reassure him and let him know that he should relax because he has got nothing to do with it. You love and accept him as he is. I do not know if he will not suffer anymore but one thing I am sure of is that this action will definitely help him against that harmful experience and this is the best you can do at that particular moment. But you have to be relaxed, aware and open-minded in order to create the right conditions.

Today is your opportunity to be conscious. Do take advantage of the information presented to you through these lines. There is no need to put a "good" or "bad" mother label on you. Always remember: *a mother is a mother*. The duality or polarity is present in our everyday life and you cannot escape it. The fight between good and bad is eternal, but the presence of unconditional love can make you aware of many things that were previously hidden behind the curtain.

One of the first few questions asked when a woman informs someone about pregnancy is this: "is it a boy or a girl?" Can you select the gender of your baby? Of course one cannot. It is impossible. We cannot choose the baby's gender, skin, hair or eye colour, nor determine its height or profession. We cannot control destiny. Perhaps, one day genetic science might be able to manipulate the human genome to create "designer babies" that will be like conditioned, beautiful robots with little or no human feelings. Thankfully, we have not got to that stage and the selection of a baby's sex remains a completely natural process. Sometimes we think that we can control nature but in the end we realize that we have done more damage than good. We want to live freely in our lives and often find ourselves saying and listening to the sentences such as *"freedom is my birthright"*. But how many babies are really born with complete freedom? Freedom in this sense means for babies to be truly free, they do not have to pass through the conditions imposed on them by their parents or others during pregnancy. I would say that the chance of a baby being born free of conditions might be around 0.0000000001%. Before the baby is even formed, we have an image or an idea about its gender. Maybe the father wants a daughter but the mother holds a different wish. Or, maybe, they start betting on its gender. Let us say one of them wins. Whose side should the baby be, father's or mother's? Surely, one of them has to be disappointed because the baby has to be one sex as he cannot be both sexes at once. I have not done any investigation on this, as I have never had a case where the baby was born a hermaphrodite. In my opinion, this can be one of the causes too. Unpleasantly and not unfortunately (because I cannot judge because if I judge then I cannot do any therapy), I have been a witness to many cases where the mother wanted to give birth to a boy but instead had a girl; so, during her childhood and youth, she participated in more boyish activities to please her mother. On the other hand, in cases where mother wanted a girl but had a baby boy, the boy wore girl's dresses and played with dolls. Nevertheless, some people might say, what is wrong with boys playing with dolls? I would say that there is nothing wrong if he freely chooses to play with dolls; however, if he is forced by some unconscious anxiety to look for mother's acceptance by playing with dolls, then his adult life could also be indirectly affected. I have not investigated this issue, but I strongly believe that homosexuality could also be one of the consequences of these preconceived ideas or thoughts about baby's gender.

The child knows without knowing what love is because he can perceive it from his mother. He just cannot define the word "love" as an adult would define it. He cannot explain it, narrate it or interpret it because he is living the experience of love. He might not know that this is an emotion, a sentiment or something else that unites him with his mother and rest of the family. But he really feels that this is a comforting sensation, an acceptance and not a rejection, togetherness and not a separation, breath and not suffocation. He is ready to live that celebration for the rest of his life, now with his mother and later with others. He is living the ecstasy of joyfulness and every cell in his being stores that valuable information. His whole life experience will depend upon what he receives during those moments. He is completely relaxed and free, flowing and growing, living in that small paradise and at the same time being grateful to his mother, to God and maybe to his own benign luck. With these celestial feelings he is ready to continue his journey to existence.

No mother is a bad mother and you should never dwell on this idea in your mind because all mothers are good and are representations of God. No mother is perfect as nobody ever is, or would ever be, or need to be. Every mother is as human as everyone else. Every mother makes mistakes as all humans do. Every mother has lived in different circumstances and had different experiences than other mothers; hence, all pregnancies are different. Every mother laughs and suffers, feels good or bad, feels calm or nervous, loves or hates, gets angry or smiles during pregnancy as she does rest of her life like all humans do. So enjoy your pregnancy. Try to live as much as possible following sentiments, emotions, feelings and experiences with your baby and always remember that above anything else, you are first and foremost, a human being. You cannot control everything and you are never responsible for everything. Sometimes circumstances are out of your control and you are forced to take certain decisions that are the best for you at that particular moment. You can repeat the titles of these sentences with your baby during pregnancy as many times as you want and the baby feels good and accepted.

"I love you unconditionally"

Unconditional love in intrauterine life is love without boundaries. It has no limits and it is unchanging. It is a form of complete love without judgement. It is infinite and immeasurable. It is given freely and it is maintaining the thought of accepting the baby as it comes. The mother should not desire or form any strong opinions about the baby. I have heard some people saying, "Oh, I want my baby to be a Taurus, Gemini or Leo because I get along well with them". "He or she should be born in summer and not in winter." "When he comes, he will be company for me because I feel lonely". All these thoughts can create difficulties during baby's birth or later in its adult life.

"I accept you as a human being that you are."

Unconditional love accepts you for the person you are and does not want to change you into someone else's idea of a person. One of the deepest needs of the human heart is the need to be valued. Everybody desires to be accepted for who he is. Nothing in human history has had such long-lasting, disastrous effects as the experience of not being accepted. When I am not accepted, then something in me is shattered. An unaccepted baby is ruined at the seed level of his existence. Everybody has that right in his life to live in unconditional love. In the intrauterine life, the baby needs to feel and live this through its mother. How amazing is it to live that whole experience again during the therapeutic session when someone had that acceptance in his or her mother's womb.

"I will completely support you and I will always be there for you no matter what."

Unconditional love is unique and beyond any doubt, word or thought. When somebody loves you without any conditions, you feel it immediately and it seems that life is beautiful and you are complete. The security of having the complete support in my life by my parents led me to do things that I never thought I could. It helped me to take right decisions even when there was nothing left in my life and I hit rock bottom. Your baby needs your support. Be there for him; make him feel loved every moment of his life. Regardless of whether you are in a pregnant state, or whether he is an adult, just show him and make him live your unconditional support as much as possible. It is the same feeling as having God's support with us round-the-clock. The mother has to practice the same thought patterns in her mind.

"You are unique and different from others and I agree that you come to this world as you are."

Unconditional love accepts you with errors because making a mistake is a part of the process towards evolution. Every person has equal right to believe, feel, do and say the things because that is his personal experience. Likewise, parents should not impose their ideas on the baby to become something or do something that they want him/her to do in life. It creates more pressure, which could later turn into a black hole in his life. He came into this life with his own purpose and has his own experiences to go through. Accept him or her as is; like everybody else, he/she is unique and different. I can never be you and you can never be me, but still we can love and respect each other.

"I do not know what is better for you or what you need and in what amount of time. Only you know this in your heart, and I can feel that my heart is connected with your heart through love."

Unconditional love brings a realization that there are many different ways of perceiving and experiencing our world, and that they are all valid. In your own life perhaps, there are some who want you to perceive life from their point of view. If you struggle with living and understanding your own experiences and depend upon them, then you will suffer low self-esteem and lack an ability to make decisions. Furthermore, you may create dependence on others and then seek their approval. Do you want your baby to experience that?

"I will totally be by your side regardless of the ideas you may have in and about life, so that you may live peacefully and comfortably."

Unconditional love is received as is in its natural form. It will freely evolve the way it is meant to. The feeling of love for someone without the need of being rewarded is different from the feeling of any other form of love. A mother should not transmit her ideas about what profession her baby should undertake; she ought to politely but firmly reject similar opinions and ideas from others. Many have suffered a great deal when they were not allowed to study the profession they wanted in life, and consequently it has affected them directly or indirectly.

On hearing other people's opinions about her child's profession, a mother could respectfully respond, "I think that we should wait to see what our baby wants to be in future and we will act accordingly." Later on, you can talk to your baby to disregard the opinions and guide it to enjoy its time in your womb.

"O divine spark, I welcome you because I know you have come to find your own individual way of relating to this world."

Unconditional love has no conditions, no judgements and it is never results-oriented. Generally speaking, your entire life is lived with conditions, judging others and is always concerned with achieving goals and objectives. That leads you to live within a constantly stressed state, which creates many negative thought patterns. The moment you become conscious of your thoughts, you allow yourself to be present and to live in freedom to be yourself. The relationship you create with your baby in his intrauterine life will form the basis of how he will relate with the world. It is like learning the language he is going to use to communicate with the outside world.

"It is a commitment that you become only what you want to be and I will be your support until you can stand on your own."

Love without conditions helps the baby live the sentiment of his real self. The mother's constant approach to support her baby leads him to live his life with confidence and find solutions to everyday problems. The parent's dedication to guide him with love to find his own path is one of the spiritual tasks of unconditional love. He will be grateful to you for everything and for all that love and care, even when you are not around. I can assure you about this with absolute confidence because I live that sentiment almost every moment of my life.

"I know that just as the way I love you, likewise I will be loved because I reap what I sow."

Did you get the freedom to become what you wanted to be? Or do you perhaps harbour regrets because you could not pursue your wishes and dreams? The affection you receive from your parents, the same you will forward to your kids, and so the cycle continues. Today is your opportunity to become conscious of your emptiness with which you lived in your childhood and seek some kind of professional help to change those negative patterns. Would you do it for you and your children? It is your decision.

"I understand that in order to do different things in different forms we need different persons."

We are all different in nature but nevertheless we are connected and dependent on each other. Our different thoughts, experiences, imaginations and actions have helped us to get to where we are today. I think that as a mother you can live the experience of demonstrating respect and understanding toward all faiths, so that one day we might also live and experience complete human understanding. The wars fought and animosity created in the name of religion would start to disappear. Unconditional love unites but it separates too. It unites us to respect and live together; it separates us because every human being needs his own space and time. In this separation there is unity and in unity there is separation. Different nationalities, customs, religions, beliefs and languages are blessings to us and we can learn to take advantage of this rich diversity in our daily lives.

Unconditional love teaches you how abundant and astonishing a mother you are. The role of mother is one of the most sanctified one from the moment a baby begins to inhabit her womb.

Some thoughts to consider

1) I know that God has chosen me to be your mother and I cannot pronounce any judgement on the experiences you are going to have. This is just my point of view and yours can be different than mine because I know that you are guided by infinite consciousness like I am.

2) Need is the basis of our existence. Our basic needs mainly consist of food, clothing, air, and shelter. But our life becomes inferior to animals if we do not love and others do not love us. The need for love is as important as breathing and water. A lack of love can create physical and mental disorders, which renders life not worth living.

3) People live their lives based on conditions. If my wife or husband does such and such, he or she loves me. Should any or some of these acts are missing, then I do not love you. There is no need to complete the requisites for the "Love Contract." The "love form" should not contain all of the necessary documents so that you can experience love successfully. Failing to submit any of the documents can delay acceptance or approval of your application. No exceptions. Can this be called love?

4) Unconditional love does not promise everything and promises everything at the same time. Although I cannot predict my behaviour and assure my control over things, I can always accept you and love you beyond everyone and everything. This is how we receive God's love. Even much before the moments your spirit arrives during the spiritual union of mother's cell with the father's, I know

you. I have known everything about you, now and always. I have always accepted you and at the same time I have always loved you unconditionally, the way you are, you think, behave, react, cry, smile, relax, sleep, work, feel good or bad, no matter what, I have always loved you and I am always there for you any time, any moment and at any place.

5) Unconditional love teaches us to be now and here. To live in present is as important as breathing. Past cannot be changed or controlled anymore and future is uncertain. Living in this very moment and feeling the emotion or celebration of unconditional love is a divine spiritual experience beyond duality. It is the experience of God loving us.

6) Unconditional love is based on feeling of living, and loving. There is no need to think about it or talk about it. Love cannot be written, read, spoken or learnt. It is there, inside you wanting to come out—like a baby wanting to take birth to meet its parents. There is no need for anybody's permission. There is no need for somebody to guide you or allow you to love. Just be love and be guided by yourself. Just do it.

7) Unconditional love is an understanding. It is an understanding of self and everybody around you. When you love yourself, then you can understand yourself. When you understand yourself, then you can also understand others. When you understand others, you can also love yourself. There is no argument in love. It is a repetitive cycle, loving and understanding and understanding and loving. It is a continuous action of life.

8) Unconditional love is limitless. When you put boundaries on love, you allow doubt to creep in. The fear of losing love becomes predominant, and your continuous cycle stops, or at least, it does not complete its revolution. At this time

meditation is required. Meditation is required to understand the obstacle. There is something new to experience and once you become aware of it, you understand how to deal with the obstacle. This is how you grow spiritually.

9) Unconditional love is an awareness of loving a human being. Loving you, your family, your neighbours, your city, your country and your planet and everything and everybody. It shows us the pathway to love God and His creation.

10) It teaches you to share with others without conditions. Everything comes to an end. Nothing is permanent. Even life is not permanent. We need to love here and now. This is the only moment available to love. There is no black, white or gray. There is no tomorrow and there was no yesterday either. There is only love. Unconditional love loves everything and everybody unconditionally. His only nature is to love and love. Everything is rooted in love. This is "God loving us and us loving God."

There is no such thing as a bad mother, for without her,
we would not be here today.
Nothing is perfect and everything is perfect.
Atul Mehra

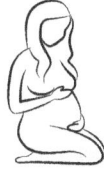

Chapter 6

"Mom, I am in your womb"
The First Button

The basis of our security and existence depends upon the love, acceptance and touch we feel in the intrauterine life; this further forms the foundation of our existence and of a balanced life. The physical and mental characteristics are transferred from parents to children in the form of biological and emotional information, including desires, inspiration, fears, happiness, frustration, expectations, etc. Nevertheless, there is no such thing as 100% acceptance, nor is there such a thing as 100% shortfall in a person's life. Hidden beneath that neurotic mask there is always an adequately healthy but unrecognized part of the self.

The basis of our lifetime is created with the intrauterine processes lived by us during the gestational nine months. The development of our eighteen senses is just the beginning, and our experiences in our mother's womb are set to determine our future. All of the information in every second is being recorded. All experiences lived by the mother are lived by the baby also. Those experiences, irrespective of whether they are good or bad, are now a natural way of connecting with the mother. In his future life, the baby needs to either live or attract the same situations that he experienced during his intrauterine life because this is now his unconscious way of connecting with his mother.

During difficult times when both mother and baby feel the pain of rejection, guilt, or abandonment, mother is able to understand and rationalize these feelings; however, the baby cannot understand the nature of what he is experiencing. He does not as yet have a rational brain to grasp the significance of his feelings. The child lives in a state of deep hypnosis for up to first three years of his life. The development of the logical-analytical mind starts later than that. These painful intrauterine experiences may become transformed and expressed later as sentiments of worthlessness, guilt, seeking attention, pleasing others, or lacking self-love.

Werner Meinhold discovered and named the intrauterine life as the "Symbiosis Phase". He explains the symbiosis phase as the foundation of a house upon which the remainder of our life's building will be constructed. In order to understand this in a more open manner, I presume to use an example from the famous German Poet Goethe who, in one of his poems, said, "if the first button of the shirt is placed into a wrong button hole then all other buttons will be wrongly placed." If a baby experiences continuous situations of conditional love, rejection and life threatening circumstances in his intrauterine life, then his life is more likely to suffer more opposition than those who have experienced more pleasant situations.

Conception happens before symbiosis. The state of consciousness is a very deep state of hypnosis. The reunion of mother and father can be perceived including acceptance and rejection between them. In order to accept myself I need to accept my parents as they are, without wanting to change them. During some therapy sessions, some of my clients experienced moments of their conception phase, which enabled them to "see" their parents in a sexual intercourse. Although they did not show any interest in that activity, they eagerly waited for the unification of an egg and a sperm so that they could take birth. They were able to perceive the emotions lived by their parents, whether it was anxiety, violence or love, acceptance, etc.

According to Meinhold, the symbiosis phase starts shortly after conception and integrates slowly with the commencement of the "oral phase" which begins after birth. Everything we need, yearn for or desire is reduced to a connection of love. On the surface this looks very simple, but it is extraordinarily difficult because it is not just a want of love, but rather a continuous effort towards total and unconditional love that we seek from the moment we come into existence. Living an incomplete intrauterine life means not being able to live and integrate healthy conditions of acceptance. This can cause psychological and physical disturbances. The experience of being accepted or loved without condition establishes a basic existential assurance. Every life has a right to exist by the mere fact of being. Generally, we do not experience this well and therefore, we do not firmly establish security in life or a state of being that leads us to unconditional acceptance. The lack of acceptance, conscious or subconscious, creates deficiencies and anxieties that are then transmuted to future life conditions. A mother who transmits her anxiety onto the baby has learned this from *her* mother. In such conditions any sound therapy would neither generate guilt nor would it change the past conditions; instead, it would aim to lead the client towards acceptance with a holistic understanding.

During this beginning period the cells multiply at dizzying and dramatic speed, organizing to form long and complicated systems of human life. The most productive period occurs during the first two months of gestation when a complete miniature human being is formed. This is the end of embryo stage and the beginning of the fetus stage, which continues to grow to a slow rhythm. The emotional stresses felt during this period generate a record of memorized reactions for rest of his life. As a developing human, he creates the neuronal-specific connections between the origins of his reactions and future events, which he will slowly but continually strengthen.

Investigation shows that depression and intrauterine fears create certain disturbances in the immune system, synapses, and the receptors of neurotransmitters, and in some cases within the brain structure. The cerebral cortex of the baby is thicker and is better equipped to learn quickly and has a highly-developed intelligence if his mother was privileged enough to live in a healthy environment where calmness, playing games, singing, and patting prevailed.

The experiences recorded during emotional traumas persist in an indelible way and may affect the cells and its functions. They remain hidden within the limbic system—the storehouse of our archaic emotional memory. This area is not naturally accessible to our developed consciousness. These stored impressions are responsible for multiple disturbances within our hormone and immune secretions. Stressful events stimulate these symbolic shortfalls, creating physical and mental discomfort, depression or even disease.

The basic anxieties borne out of rejection ensure that these rejected parts of the personality are routed and suppressed into the unconsciousness. Here they reside and become the roots of self-injurious and self-destructing psychosomatic disease. The "bad" or deficient parts of the personality can turn into malignant disease. Disease is simultaneously an expression of trauma as well as of the security of existence (being) through which the person expresses himself. Insisting on removing these deficient parts of personality could cause malignancies through morbid metastasis. When the symbiotic phase is disturbed, we cannot perceive life as an expression of the essence, and therefore, it exists with complete right and security by itself.

A great majority of diseases and disturbances that appear to be related to one or more of the early development periods have their origin (or, the first button hole) in the symbiosis phase. The phase where disturbance is generally found shows the intent to compensate the lack of basic existential security. If the baby did not feel the experience of initial acceptance he will use the rest of his life to fill this lack, but as this is not the respective buttonhole to that button, he will never resolve the feeling of not having received it at its due time. For example, even though I can do everything, I am never satisfied.

If the moments of birth are problematic then it means that already there were problems in the symbiotic phase. If there is a premature delivery or if the baby does not want to take birth at this time then there has to be a reason behind it.

During my research, I came across two beautiful excerpts describing the symbiosis phase and I take this opportunity to share it with you. Both of them connected me with my own experiences with intrauterine life and also reveal that different experiences at different times with different people can lead us to the same results. What I really like about Dr. Liley's explanation of intrauterine life is that it is built upon his underlying belief in the unborn as a complete being from the first instance and in all of the natural processes happening in the mother's womb. I accept and agree completely based on my knowledge and experience. He clearly explains the sense of self, the sense of movement and sense of freedom.

Dr. William A. Liley, also known as the "Father of Fetology", described the intrauterine phase thus:

"The young individual, in command of his environment and destiny with a tenacious purpose, implants in the spongy or endometrial wall of the womb and, with a remarkable display of physiologic power, suppresses his mother's menstrual period. This will be his home for the next 270 days and to make it habitable, the embryo develops a placenta and a protective amniotic fluid capsule for him. We know that fetus is always moving in its exuberant world, and that fetal comfort determines fetal position. He is responsive to pain and touch, cold, sound and light. He feeds himself with his amniotic fluid; he absorbs more, if it's artificially sweetened and a less quantity if it does not like the taste. He sobs and sucks his thumb. He wakes and sleeps. He does not like the repetitive signals but he can be taught to distinguish two successive signals. And, finally, he determines the day of his birth, because, without any doubt, the onset of labor is a unilateral decision of the unborn. This is the fetus we know, and one day each one of us was. This is the fetus we look after in modern obstetrics, the same baby we are caring for before and after birth and before seeing the light of the day he can get sick and needs diagnosis and treatment just like any other patient."

The second one is a letter written by Claude Imbert addressed to future parents, one that illustrates the principles of love and unconditional acceptance...

"We babies need our conception to be focused on our good and our harmony. For us to receive this choice of life, besides thinking about us as embryos and foetuses, think that we are conceived for ourselves in the best available time and love, desired and expected without condition."

"We are created in our mother's womb through a fusion of egg and sperm, at the same time in their minds and especially in their hearts. It is this loving energy that feeds and sustains us far beyond the umbilical cord, providing us with nutrients our bodies need to grow. This is a virtual channel, one so strong that it can deliver

love to every cell, to the very core of our being so that we may become complete in our development."

"At the moment of our creation, we expect to receive love and wisdom. It is as if our whole future depends on it, all our thoughts, emotions, actions and reactions of our future life center on the presence of this love. It gives us untold strength, makes us powerful within, and allows us to move mountains in future. What seem to us as insurmountable obstacles, discouragements, sadness, feelings of incapacity, fears of all kinds, will now be understood and resolved."

"Everything is possible within this powerful force of love. This is what we expect of you, if you choose to be the actors that allow our creation. We hope that the seed is implanted not only in the womb of our mother, but also in your minds and especially in your hearts. We hope that your characteristics change upon becoming parents, and at the same time you enable circumstances so that we may evolve as we enter into this world."

I consider both of them as the classic true masterpieces for our knowledge and progress.

Now going beyond that materialistic perception of intrauterine life, I consider that the baby's life itself is a complete life cycle in the intrauterine period. He lives a complete human life during pregnancy. He decides to be in the mother's womb. He starts waking up slowly and develops organs that would later be indispensable for him. It is a happy time for the embryo as the simple form of a chrysalis extends around him, the membrane that serves as protection and liquid that envelops and feeds him. He lives freely and collects the natural wisdom of learning, which later will determine the shape of his body and the unique features of his face. This phase is known as the blessed childhood of an embryo.

Immediately after comes the adolescence of the fetus, the human form is perfected and the sex is determined. The placenta that makes up the external body of the fetus feels that some unknown force is growing within it and is driven to break and escape from it. His brain reflects his mother's like a mirror image. By then, the mother is for the baby what God is for us, i.e., an entity unknown and invisible. Mother is like God to the baby growing in her womb. The embryo tends to her, lives thanks to her, but cannot see or seem to understand her. If he could philosophize, he would possibly deny the personal existence and the intelligence of his mother. Up until then, his mother's womb was a lethal prison and the object of his perception.

Next comes the adult stage of the baby where all his body parts are developed and his intelligence and awareness are at their peak as far as intrauterine life goes. He reacts to the soft or painful moments in this environment and begins to acquire information and experiences through his body parts and emotions. He lives in communion with his mother and experiences everybody and everything through her.

Bit by bit, this bondage causes him discomfort and he moves, suffers, feels tormented and thinks that his life is at an end. When he is overcome with maximum distress and tremors, his bonds come unleashed and he feels as though he is falling into the abyss of the unknown. Suddenly, he feels painful sensations that make him shudder. A strange coldness enters his space, and he inhales his last breath in the womb. As he exhales this breath, it transforms into his first cry as a newborn. The intrauterine life is transformed into human life.

*Communication is felt only if hearts
are joined together.*
Atul Mehra

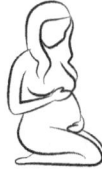

Chapter 7

Mother and Baby Communication

I left India in my early 20s in order to travel and explore the world. I recall receiving a letter from my family after months of waiting and then reading it as many times as possible. I carried it in my pocket for days and felt the love, connection, warmth and emotional support from it that enabled me to overcome the challenges I later faced in various foreign countries. Even today I feel a longing for those memory imprints.

I felt a telepathic connection with my family and with those who have been very near to me. It still surprises me to this day when I experience the sensations and information beyond the limits of time and distance. Sometime I wish I go back to those times and feel and live those sensations to my fullest.

I am certain that many of you have lived similar moments many times in your life and have memories that transport you back to those times. While writing this I am also reminded of song lyrics that still create a feeling of nostalgia; in India, I had acted in an opera called "Joseph And The Amazing Technicolor Dream

Coat" and sang the lyrics "*Those Canaan days we used to know, where have they gone, where did they go? Eh bien, raise your berets to those Canaan days.*"

The sense of connection is associated with these memories and a simple idea or imagination of a part triggers sensations of warmth, love, and acceptance. This is the experience of communication that will stay with me forever. Unfortunately, the cell phones and other electronic devices are slowly destroying our receptor organ responsible for this kind of communication, the pineal gland.

When I return to the present day, I begin to wonder, "What happened? Why do I feel differently? Why do I not have the same intense sensations when I receive a message or talk to them? In fact, we have become so habituated and dependent on modern technology that we have begun acting like automatons. There is less communication now because people are becoming socially isolated. I don't want to deviate from the topic besides all of you know this modern issue very well. However, we now know that not only do they undoubtedly affect us, but also the fact that they can impact the future of a baby for the rest of his life. This is to the extent that many of the physical or psychological ailments suffered by an adult can have their origin in something that occurred while he was in his mother's womb.

If I asked someone in this present time to name the different types of communication systems that exist, he would probably answer in materialistic terms, '4' and first would be written which includes magazines, books, emails, written letters, etc. The second would be oral which is both speaking and listening. The third one would be non-verbal which is connected to body gestures, and finally, visual communication which is everything that our physical eyes can see. But I would certainly add *telepathic* or *direct* communication to that list. It means that the baby is directly absorbing any form of communication that reaches the mother.

Many years ago a client came to me in her quest to lose weight. She was doing everything: dieting, exercising, taking weight-reduction tablets, but nothing was working. She had a long scar that was like a line on her cheek. She explained that she was born with a big, black spot on her face that made her feel uncomfortable throughout her childhood. She had low self-esteem and did not accept herself. This resulted in an unhealthy environment in which to grow up. When she became an adult, she underwent an operation to remove the black spot, but unfortunately, the long scar remained on her face. She came to the session with her sister who was 5 years older than her. During the session she accessed the memory of being in her mother's womb and discovered that when she was approximately 3 months' old, her mother went to see a lady who revealed that her thigh had a very nasty spot. Her mother felt disgusted and nauseated.

This client describes, "I am scared, my mother feels very badly, my hands and feet are very small, I cannot have that spot there but my face is bigger." Now that was the moment when a malignant black spot was created on her face and she carried for a long time even after birth. She further discloses the connection between not losing weight and this experience. After finishing the session when she shared her experience with her sister, she confirmed, "Yes, I remember as I was 5 years old. I was with Mom and after that mother felt sickened and vomited." Then they went to see that lady as if a kind of secret was revealed in her life. Up until this day, I am still curious to know what exactly happened there and how that spot was formed. I could not do more sessions to inquire more as I was there only for some time. I thought to share it with you so that you could understand and become aware of the role communication plays in pregnancy.

In order to make this topic understandable, I would simply divide the topic of Mother-Baby communication during pregnancy in two categories: the **Conscious** and the **Unconscious** communication.

Conscious communication consists of everything that is consciously done by the mother during her pregnancy. During this communication she communicates with the baby in a healthy manner, such as singing, talking, loving and accepting her baby completely with the participation of father. In the second category of conscious but unhealthy communication are such things such as rejecting the baby, creating conditions about her gender, drinking/smoking or taking recreational drugs knowingly.

The unconscious communication consists of what happens beneath the surface and the mother is unaware of it. It can include previous healthy or unhealthy pregnancies, love bonds or arguments with husband, being scared while watching horror movies or laughing at comedies, conditional or unconditional conversations about pregnancies, or any thought, imagination, perception with strong emotions attached to them can also influence the development of the baby. Baby communicates through kicking and movement. For example, when his mother sings or he likes a particular type of music, he may move or kick the mother softly, but when he is exposed to loud noise or an unpleasant event, then he may revolt against it with a series of painful kicks or strong, painful movements. I remember during the time when my second daughter was in her mother's womb, I asked her which movie she wanted to see and on saying the first one, she moved softly but she also moved when I asked her about the second one. I think the movie was irrelevant to her as long as she was being taken into consideration and knowing that she was part of a family event; this is the pathway to feeling loved and accepted.

I could have written many complicated details about this topic but my idea was to keep it as simple as possible. In order to understand it in a simpler way I would like to share an example. When you get up early in the morning and you say, "Today is going to be an excellent day." What do you think would happen? What if you say, "Today is going to be a terrible, rotten day." What do you think would happen? We attract good or bad events based on the quality of our ideas or thoughts. If we remain positive, we will be able to handle negative events in a better way. A positive thought is not enough but a continuous positive process is. I think that there is already so much information available in this book that it is sufficient to consider and understand many things about communication. I always say, "Life is simple, don't make it complicated and also pregnancy is simple; just enjoy it, be positive, accept your baby, laugh, take care of your health and use common sense. Everything is going to be all right. Do not be anxious about anything because anxiety attracts." Meinhold says that anxiety and desire are one and the same. If you have anxiety that this could happen, then you have a desire that this should happen. Pregnancy ought to be a celebration of new life, and not regarded as torturous. If the circumstances in your life are less than satisfactory, then please postpone your plan of having a baby. If you are not ready then it means you are not ready and it is as simple as that.

What affects your health affects the health of the baby as well. When something makes you feel good and wanted, the baby feels and lives it too. You are the captain of your "pregnancy" ship and you can navigate to calm waters or you can rollick in stormy seas. It is your choice. This is not rocket science; in fact, it is very straight and simple. Drugs, tobacco, alcohol, depression, arguments, fighting, feeling badly, and negative emotions are not good for health in general, especially during pregnancy. On the other hand laughing, exercising, yoga, meditation, love, kindness, feeling good and positive emotions are all good for health and will result in a healthy pregnancy.

In the baby lies the future of the world. Mother must hold the baby close so that the baby knows it is his world but the father must take him to the highest hill so that he can see what his world is like.
Mayan Proverb

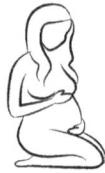

Chapter 8

"Dad Loves Me Too"
The Role of the Father

Osho once said that when a baby is born, a mother is also born. I would strongly assert that when a baby is born, not only is a mother born, but also so is a father. Although it is the mother who carries the baby for nine months, the father's active participation in the process right from preconception onwards is of equal importance and value. The father's regular visits to the doctor with the mother and his presence during the time of birth goes a long way in helping to build a healthy pregnancy. These connections forged with the baby during pregnancy become the blueprints for the rest of its life.

I read somewhere once and I paraphrase it here: "World can live without a father but not without a mother. Father is a social obligation which we will have to carry." For years this statement haunted me, leaving me feeling confused and burdened by guilt – as a future father, would I be simply perceived as a social obligation and nothing else? In my own experience, my father was my master, my teacher, plus so much more. That statement created a subconscious disturbance within me, indirectly affecting an integral part of me. Whenever I witnessed a father disciplining his children, I became acutely aware of my sensitivity to his role as a father and judged it as not being the right way to treat children. Clearly, I was under the influence of my faulty interpretations and thoughts that arose out of that statement stated previously. Perhaps guided at a subconscious level, years later, I was to experience a father's role when our first baby was born. It was only then that I realized that a father is not a social obligation; rather, he occupies a very special place in a baby's life. The baby can feel a father's presence or absence while it is still in the mother's womb, a feeling that can deeply impact his life. During my whole life therapy process through integrated therapy of Depth Psychology under hypnosis, I underwent this amazing experience as I felt my father's presence and his love while I was in my mother's womb. Those unconscious bonds with my parents became more conscious and helped me to remove the load of anxieties, fears and preconceived filters which could have easily led me to divorce, dissatisfaction, and poor mental health. Instead, this experience freed me to receive and process the information so that I could live my life more freely.

We cannot love ourselves in parts; we must accept our whole body to become complete. Similarly, a baby is incomplete without its mother and its father. A baby acquires its DNA from both parents. Although a unique and separate human being, a baby inherits his parents' genetic traits that become imprinted into his personality traits. If there is conditional acceptance then those parts remain unrecognized, and sooner or later, they express themselves through a disorder or a disease. However, this is still considered to be a healthy expression from the body's point of view. The human body has the innate wisdom to seek and create not only a symptom but also to heal it completely. The way to resolve this issue depends upon finding the correct therapeutic pathway. Regrettably, many times there are circumstances when a baby is abandoned for whatever reason. The father could not be with the baby for whatever reason, and therefore had to be absent from his life. The baby feels a great sense of fear, abandonment and loneliness, which may manifest later in life in a similar way when he lives apart from his own children. Therapeutically, these issues can be resolved, however, in some cases it may take a bit longer.

There are situations where a father does not recognize or see his son. Over time, the son creates a telepathic connection with father and takes on his personality traits. You might have heard someone saying something like this: "You are just the same as your father, even though you've never met him."

Sometimes when the mother has issues with the father, she might think and speak ill of him. This information is retained by the baby and may indirectly affect his life. It can happen during pregnancy or even during early childhood. The baby is not responsible for the problems between his mom and dad. Witnessing arguments between mom and dad, whether during pregnancy or in childhood, a baby may hold himself responsible for them and feel obligated to choose sides. In particular, while in-vitro, the baby is bound to feel the same as his mother, creating a psychological resistance to completely accepting the father.

We cannot ignore the role of the father during pregnancy. Do you remember those times past when fathers would be sent outside the birthing room to wait while the midwife tended to the woman in labour? In some parts of the world there is a persistent belief that the father cannot be present in the birthing room because he could transmit some sort of an infection that could be harmful to the baby. I cannot judge this belief or practice because I have experienced it. During the birth of my first daughter, I decided to be with my wife when her water was broken. We worked as a team to manage her labour pain through breathing exercises. I remember putting on a medical white overcoat, a head cover, mouth cover, and shoes so that I would not transmit any germs or infection to risk the baby's health. The gynecologist was covered in a similar manner. I can still feel those beautiful, warm sensations when I first set eyes on my baby daughter. After cutting the umbilical cord, the Doctor showed me the bloody placenta and humorously remarked that I might be too scared to see the blood. Instead, I jokingly replied "You had better take it back home with you and put it in front of the main entrance so no vampire would dare come in." We laughed over this, and after that I assured my newborn daughter that everything is alright and that they were going to take her someplace for a short while but soon she would be with us again.

Now, in any other medical facility people would have viewed this exchange as insane; however, our gynecologist was very open-minded and knew of my work in the field of psychology. He knew that my concern was to ensure that my daughter did not feel any kind of fear of separation. I still vividly recall those tender moments when I followed her outside that room as the nurse placed her behind a big glass wall. I went close against the wall made the same sounds as when she was in the womb. When I called her name, she moved her head to look at me and immediately I felt as though it was the most miraculous moment of my life. It was such a divine feeling that even as I write these lines, I feel my eyes welling up. Who would not like to experience such cherished moments in their life?

My second daughter was born in Canada, but this time I was not asked to wear anything for her protection. Her birth also went smoothly. Being the second time around, I was better prepared for the process. I respectfully agreed with all the things doctors advised us to do during pregnancy, however, I discreetly did all the things I knew to do in order to avoid complications at birth. Throughout this time, I remained in synchronization with my daughter. The doctor suggested that my wife have a surgery should she not deliver the baby at the expected time. I was so sure about my experience that I decided to wait until the next two days as the pregnancy App suggested (the mobile app suggested the date 17 for her birth as I was also born on 17 and my interest in numerology made me like the idea and also we discussed many times the same date during pregnancy and I knew that my daughter was listening). My wife felt the labour pains, and I stayed beside her until it was time to deliver the baby. I am sure that she was conscious and aware of her birth, as she did not cry for some time. There is a very deep symbolism connected with the baby's first cry. Doctors say that babies cry immediately after birth because it helps their lungs to breathe. In depth psychology we know that every separation is painful. A baby cries because he separates from his mother. In Catholicism, man's sin results in a separation from God.

I knew that we shared a telepathic communication, so when the nurse shared that information with me about crying, I felt that it would be better if she cried, and within moments she started crying! During the in-vitro time of my second daughter, I experienced many memories and emotions from my own childhood that made me feel deeply connected. I consider myself very fortunate to have had these blessed and wonderful experiences with my daughters. I would never fail to remind others to not miss out on this once-in-a-lifetime opportunity.

The discovery of paternal power was very illuminating. The father's intention also exerts a huge impact on the baby's intention to live and to develop. The main emotion to feel here for the baby is that he is desired and wanted by both Mom and

Dad. I communicated with both my daughters during my wife's pregnancies and assured them every now and then that everything was all right, and more so during times when we would argue over something over some vague problem in our household. Both of them heard my voice during and after pregnancy, guiding them until they became aware of themselves. I frequently recall the advice my own father used to impart to me in the form of rhymes when I was quite young. Later, these songs of advice helped me during my travels across many countries and served to inspire and sustain me through rough patches, such as the time when my documents and money were stolen and I had to face many hardships.

From the moment you explore your desire to have a baby, you have the opportunity to create awareness that being more joyful and present with your partner will create conditions for a healthy pregnancy. The warmth of physical touch and affections of the heart, the gentle sexual intimacy, the tender expressions of love and other forms of unconditional acceptance are all key to a baby's good health.

We also have to take into consideration the parents' own prenatal and perinatal experiences in all of this. If their parents suffered a disturbance such as a miscarriage or any other traumatic experience during their pregnancy, then they subconsciously influence the baby with these fears. I would strongly recommend a counselling session or two to overcome that.

You may not be convinced but doctors also play a very important role in pregnancy. They have a moral obligation towards their patients in that they must be careful to select and use words carefully so that the baby does not feel rejected or threatened. Many doctors today understand this important point, yet many remain ignorant of the difficulties caused by a careless word or a remark. In a future chapter, I will be sharing "How I created my own miracle in my life." This is a case of my client whose tumour disintegrated after therapy. Interestingly, the seeds of this tumour were implanted in the mother's womb.

Now we know that the roles of the father, the mother, and the doctor play an important part in pregnancy and childbirth. So, what is the role of all those others around you – siblings, grandparents, uncles and aunts? Well, they also share this responsibility as they too can indirectly influence the baby's development.

In order to gain a deeper understanding about the role of the father, we have to first understand the symbolism of the father. The archaic symbolism of the father within the Christian context is embodied in the person of Jesus Christ. He is a very noble and gentle father of his followers. He unconditionally loves and forgives all. The Group symbolism of the Father represents the role of the protector. He goes out to work, earn, bring food home, loves his family, provides education to his children, and disciplines his children when necessary. According to individual symbolism, the father was very cruel, treated his son badly, rejected him and abandoned him. As you can see, the archaic symbol is incongruent to the Group symbol and Individual symbol. It means that there is a disease/disorder present. With an appropriate therapeutic approach, we can correct the significance of these symbolisms, turning disorder into a peaceful lesson. The truth is that if you want to have peace in your life, then make peace with your mother and father and the rest will follow naturally.

Here I will describe a case where early life experiences are seen to affect adult relationship with the father. The client gave me his permission to share his experience as a part of healthy process to find the importance of father for others.

Daniel** is 20 years old, a single male who feels lonely, is scared of snakes (masculine symbol), fears physical obstacles, accidents and death. He does not have a very good relationship with his father. He considers his father to be a very complicated person although he thinks of him as the most beloved person in his life. He also reflects that in his past, he had been the reason that he became ill. He remembered having lots of arguments with him in the past. He often felt the absence of his father as he was usually away working. These and other pathological events did not allow him to have complete awareness of his father but now things were going to change. He wanted to resolve his relationship with his father. He started his whole life therapy process under the guidelines of Integrative therapy of depth psychology as created by Werner Meinhold.

The idea of sharing this experience is to understand how our subconscious operates, and although the answers reside within us, we cannot fully access them unless we work through our issues in an integrative manner. There has to be complete openness to accept without guilt and to integrate those unrecognized parts of our personality that had remained under lock and key. As these memories remain censured for a long time, accessing them too rapidly could prove traumatic to a client. We followed a long pathway of many sessions in order to unwrap these events. The following dialogues are in a summary of few sessions together. After a full year of therapy, he arrived at the stage where he was two years old in his chronological age. He describes the following (the spoken words appear in italics):

"... I am in my house... I feel that I am in my house because I do not see it...

I asked him, *"How does that make you feel?"*

"Relaxed"…he replied, now on confirming the feeling of relaxation allows him to make him feel more secure and helps to open the memory a little bit more and he continues…

"I am climbing the stairs … there is someone who is watching me… it is a shadow"

"Who is the shadow?" I asked, he did not answer.

"How do you feel with the shadow?" I asked him again after some time.

"It makes me feel secure that it is taking care of me" … he replied …*"I feel peace, it seems that it is passing by to see me and goes away and it does not have a face… it is a shadow."*

I know that he is talking about his father but there is still a resistance to recognize him. This means that we need to devote further sessions to work through his anxiety that is preventing him from recognizing the "shadow". I cannot help him in this quest of discovering his father's face because that would be iatrogenic (Relating to illness caused by medical examination or treatment or by the healthcare professional or therapist). He has to come to this recognition on his own so that he could unveil the hidden and establish a natural bond with his father.

He continued *"I feel safe because it is looking out for me, a mother would do the same-she is in the store (Stationery shop)… I am with my Grandmother."* (Now he takes more awareness of his present situation).

"How do you feel?" I asked.

"Fine, there is no problem… but I feel alone, it is not something intense but just few moments… a little bit anxious…

sadness, sometimes I am left alone, a little bit of insecurity, I feel alone, it affects me when I feel alone, I feel anxiety to forget this loneliness ... I do not have anyone to share with but I am also not going to die because of that (he is now taking awareness and relating it with his present age of 20 years and at the same time living the experience of chronological age)... I know in a short while it is going to arrive, tomorrow I am going to convert into a person... I give time to time."

This awareness helped him to understand the underlying issues connected with his present day emotions and issues arising as a result.

He further confirms but he is still resistant to recognize, *"I feel like a protection... I am in someone's arms, holding tightly, I do not see anything, Just manage to feel...I am being hold tightly and I want to walk... when you walk, relax and move your muscles (he suggests himself).*

Interestingly, the organs of movements i.e. arms and legs are connected with the development of the sense of movement, the sense of freedom and also the sense of self which are being integrated. The session ended with him feeling security and protection, which are very important to access the memories kept under lock and key by the subconscious. Now it becomes more interesting how experiencing these feelings helps him to recognize his father on his own.

Upon feeling that security and protection, he connects with a memory of the past and recollects that he is with his grandmother and he is crying, and she says to him, *"Do not cry, your Mom and Dad are coming and they are going to feed you."* This word Dad in this sentence immediately brings his father out of the shadow and now the connection is created and the face becomes visible. During the next few sessions, he rationalizes and completes his experience with his father.

He describes his tranquility in a symbolic way at the beginning of the sentence...

-"...I feel that I am in a Sea or in the water, I only feel, it relaxes me. I feel some hands...seem to me of my Dad, they are making me sleep, they pass through the face so I feel sleepy, he is caressing me, I feel relaxation, love and it gives me lot of peace. (Now on recognizing his father he brings up memories of healthy and loving moments with his father)

He continued, "Now I see how he moves away, I don't like it...I feel restless, when he goes away then I cry, I get angry, I feel bad, and I start to cry like a crazy, I start feeling a desperate sensation...when I feel he goes away, in my heart, in my mind, in my body, it is like a 'shiver' which runs throughout my body. I don't know where he goes? I feel anxious."

Now he is taking awareness of the sensation he feels when his father goes away. Since he is in complete wakefulness, he resolves by himself that mystery with his logical analytical mind of 20 years.

-"...Every time he goes away, I understand, may be, like before he goes to work, to feed us, to his family, (Now this analytical awareness transforms that anxiety into something more beautiful and connected with father)...It makes me prouder instead of feeling worried, maybe he felt the same when he used to go to work, thus I sacrificed and he did too. May be this desperation starts there. I prefer giving him a hug before saying anything."

Now he feels and lives those hidden sensations of warmth towards his father.

-"...*There is a lot of warmth in his arms, first I feel warmth with happiness...I want to say something...this is not more than a hug, they are same, he does not care sacrificing for me...I am always going to have his support and I perceive this in his eyes before his words, this is something straight, more than names and words I see expressions and acts...I try to feel him and he is not there, I feel a kind of sorrow as I was having a good time. He goes away but I am sure that he is going to come back.*"

These are very magical moments for him and after feeling that security, creating a basic connection and reaching on to this understanding his relationship with his father changed dramatically and they both experienced a healthier relationship than before.

**"Daniel" is a fictitious name; the real name has been omitted for reasons of privacy and confidentiality.*

In another case, an adult woman re-lived the moments of her birth during our first few sessions together. She had this strong sense of her father's feelings towards her because he wanted to have a boy but she was a girl. During the session she cried and said, "*I am taking birth and everybody is surprised; my father says about me, what is this?*"

She explained after the sessions, "*I thought I had resolved everything. I have had 5 years of therapy with 14 different therapists but I never went that deep in any of my sessions. Now I know why I have less hair in this age. Now, I know why I never fed my baby from the right breast. Now, I know why I created a cancer in my right breast (symbolically right side of the body represents the father).*"

A therapeutic process is based on recognizing the union of both parts, masculine and feminine in their level of spiritual and biological energy. A client can also perceive and accept reservations, rejections or conditions of acceptance of one family member for another in order to fulfill their basic, unconscious need for love. This is seen as the sensation of the right to have the warmth of life that must be established as an exclusive property of the client, given to him as a cosmic and spiritual right. It is essential for the universe that this human take birth under these conditions. The ability to consciously accept these conditions in which this right is given to us creates an expanded awareness resulting in a state of bliss and warmth, and it is free of distress and is completely safe.

This sensation is experienced many times in life, such as the time when love is felt with great intensity between two beings, leading to a recognition or connection that "I am you or we are one." The capacity to feel and understand love in such a deep way lies within each of us. It becomes our task to develop this capacity of perceiving and expressing this unconditional acceptance of all beings. The idea is to connect with this level of consciousness since love always exists but only after we have experienced the situations that allow us to live the expansion and acknowledgement of the union between the two.

Our fears can be brought into consciousness, from almost a permanent anxiety to a panic that may shadow a pregnancy. It may be that it had existed even before conception in every sexual relationship. These fears that emanate from the mother have different causes; especially genealogical in the form of memories of pregnancies and deliveries transmitted through the family tree. These fears can be associated with serious injuries or deaths of a child or mother in different moments of gestation, neonatal period and of birth, and can be reactivated in later generations.

They may also be generated by the complications that appeared either in a preceding or a subsequent pregnancy such as hemorrhages, a spontaneous abortion, and therapeutic or voluntary interruption. In other cases, there can be a reactivation of the memories lived by the mother as a baby during her intrauterine life or at the time of her birth especially if it was a difficult one.

This fear of reproduction will cause distress, sadness, and guilt within the child, and the past limitations lived by the mother may become imprinted upon its own sexual development. If the mother feels that she is in danger, the embryo will perceive this to be the reality and will blame his existence as a threat to his mother's or his own life. A baby who lives its intrauterine life surrounded by maternal fears such as accidents during her pregnancy or accidents of past generations might perceive the male's sperm as dangerous, and consequently generate infertility or impotence in order to create a sense of security for his partner.

I am sure that those parents who have witnessed the miracle of birth will forever remember it as one of the most remarkable moments in their lives. At the same time, I would implore God to not allow any parent to witness any of the hurting or any painful childbirth experiences. God forbid, if you are amongst them and you have not been able to overcome that loss or trauma, then please write a word to me and I will do my best to help you to overcome that experience.

May God bless all the future parents and their babies.

My faith in God can die,
But God's faith in me will never die.
Atul Mehra

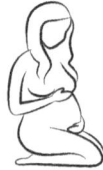

Chapter 9

And the Tumour Disintegrated

Behave yourself or I will give you my cancer. How crazy and funny this sentence would sound if we were to hear it being spoken in real! All of us want to live a healthy life. So, what exactly is health? You might say that it is being free from illness, injury or pain. Would one consider a person healthy if he/she never smoked or drank, ate a healthy diet, exercised, and took care of his health, and yet died from a heart attack at the age of 40?

The word health comes from the old English word *hal,* meaning wholeness or total. We cannot love ourselves in parts. It is ridiculous to say that I love my right arm more than my left arm, or my right leg is better than my left eye. Humans are born with body parts, organs, cells, and tissues, as well as thoughts, sentiments, and emotions. Everything that happens within me can be considered as my *self* or *being.* If I lack something within me, then this opens up an opportunity for something else to take its place.

There is no rational way in which we can plan our lives where diseases are concerned. For instance, no one consciously sets out to acquire diabetes at age 15, multiple sclerosis at age 25, cancer at age 30, or even death at age 32; and yet, we know of loved ones or friends who have been affected by these chronic illnesses resulting in death at an early age. Who or what is responsible for this? Recognizing that we create our own diseases and knowing the origin of this offers us hope so that we may find ways to restore our health and wellbeing. Whether it is cancer, diabetes, anxiety or any other disorder, the person creates it by himself at an unconscious level.

The presence of chronic diseases in one's life is always considered unfortunate. Disease is unkind and I completely support this idea that when you are sick, it is important and necessary to go to the doctor for medical treatment. As the symptoms begin to resolve through treatments, I suggest taking this opportunity to recognize the work that has just started, and dive deeper into the depths of the shadowy process of a disease.

Life starts from a single cell consciousness in the mother's womb, and, after passing through billions of processes, it culminates into the final form to become ONE or whole. From that very moment to now, these processes require the best possible unconditional growth of the self. Endless obstacles, repressions, or opposing those processes can create further mental or physical illnesses in the future.

I witnessed a miracle where I observed the emergence of those malignant energies that created a tumour. The whole life therapeutic process brought new ideas, new surprises and new experiences that concluded as an amazing event. I will now share a story of one of my clients who underwent therapy and shared her experiences related to disintegrating a tumour in her body. I have her enthusiastic and express permission to share her incredible story with you. It is incredible to me to realize that the conditions experienced in a mother's womb could also act as fertile grounds for a benign tumour to take root and grow later in her life. I will call my client Alba in order to respect her privacy and to protect her real identity.

In April 2006, Alba started yoga classes with me. She revealed that she suffered from pain in her right knee. After a few classes, we discussed and explored the symbolism related to her knee pain, and she recognized the connection and agreed to begin the whole life therapy process under hypnosis based on Dr. Werner Meinhold's techniques and guidelines. The therapeutic process ended in April 2010.

She had been under the care of a psychiatrist who was treating her for the past six months for depression and anxiety. She was hospitalized for five days to undergo sleep therapy, received weekly sessions, and took many medications (anti-psychotics and anti-depressants) for months thereafter without any improvement in her symptoms. She said, "I carried out only what the doctor told me to do because I wanted to be released from the hospital. The anxieties continued, I felt sadness inside me, I did not find any peace; moreover I could not find any solutions to what led me into this state."

She also disclosed her difficult relationship with her parents and siblings. Approximately 15 years ago, she began to experience irregular menstrual periods. Later, blood tests results detected higher prolactin and she was diagnosed with Polycystic Ovary Syndrome. Her gynecologist prescribed medications to be taken daily for the rest of her life. Eventually, a small tumour on Sella Turcica in the Pituitary gland was discovered. The most amazing part was that we always talked about her fears, resentments, anxieties, fantasies and realities, but never really openly discussed the benign tumour she had. Nor did I have much experience in this area, and thought of it as more as the domain of a medical professional or a neurosurgeon. For me, psychotherapy was a treatment for those who suffer from mental health problems. While in therapy with me, my client faithfully took her medication in order to menstruate and to manage high prolactin... until her doctor asked her to stop it completely.

I decided to write down her words because I think it is important for every one of us to understand that we create our own miracles in our life. The origin of unhealthy life lies in us and the opportunity to reverse that process depends on us too. Creating openness, the capacity to understand myself with awareness, and making peace with others as well as with myself, all have the capability of creating miracles in my life. This, of course, must be paired with facing our basic fears in an integrative manner.

We started the whole life therapy process and during our second year of therapy the tumor grew a little bit more. I remember having discussed with her and we continued the therapy; gradually, she began to make room for peace in her life. In her words...

"During these fantastic – very often, difficult and emotionally strong moments – I learned to know myself better, to accept me as I am and to love myself. I learned to look at and accept my parents and siblings as they are: human beings with successes and mistakes; I learned to look at them with love, try not to judge them but to understand them, I learned to forgive what had to be forgiven and accept what I had lived and to understand what I lived it for. It was learning at every moment, in every circumstance. During therapy, and after finishing it, I have been able to move closer to my father with love, respect and acceptance, and no longer with anger and resentment which I had felt towards him, because during the therapy, I understood many things related to his attitude towards me, and it opened my heart. I could also accept the alienation of my brother and accept it as it is, to forgive him for

not wanting to get closer to me; I understood and I stopped feeling the pain of rejection. Likewise with my mom, I could heal some resentment that I had kept very deep inside me. I started talking and moving closer to my sister with whom I had a strong conflict and we had not talked for a long time."

She continues, *"In therapy, I realized why I had to maintain stormy loving relationships. I used to harm myself by getting involved with the wrong people who hurt me and above all, I allowed them to hurt me. Based on that understanding, I was able to get away from my best friend because his friendship was not convenient, and I got the courage to say enough and think first of my own well-being, and from then onwards, I am in peace, and now I am not looking for someone to hurt me, because now I know that I only deserve to receive love and I can give love. As therapy advanced, I knew a little more of myself, I was learning to value more, to love, to understand people close to me, and how my whole environment, my beliefs* and my way of seeing and living life had influenced me to be who I was at that time."

"It is incredible to look back now on how I was a conflicted person, sometimes sad and depressed, dependent on others to take decisions, looking for others' approval, fearful to make certain decisions. Right after the therapy, I realized that I am the one who chooses which path to follow. Previously, I chose the difficult path, with sadness and despair, with suicide attempts, and with frustrations. The path which I now travel and enjoy is full of happiness, optimism, internalizing every day, living and breathing life with the open heart, with the healthy body, with an open mind and looking for new options, with more freedom of heart to love and letting others love me too. Part of that beautiful process of self-awareness led me to realize that when I was twelve years old I was very afraid of growing up, moving from girl to become a woman, for different experiences and situations that I would discover and understand as the therapy sessions advanced. All of

this led me to understand that it was that fear that made me generate prolactin problems and consequently appearance of the tumour in the pituitary gland. This great understanding led me to the healing process, I understood and accepted my fears, embraced them, forgave myself and moved ahead, and to the surprise of my attending physician, the tumour disappeared, my prolactin stabilized and I stopped taking medication."

"I remember the time after the exams, my treating doctor saw the results and was surprised. He said that for him there was no other reason than a miracle, because it was one in a million case that the tumor disappeared and everything became normal in such a short time. He could not accept my theory that the work on my self-awareness helped me to heal, but he told me that he is not completely ruling out that possibility...Since the time the test results were positive until now, ten years have passed, and my body works very well, I have regular periods without the use of medicines."

I shared this testimonial with you because I think it is a call to awaken our consciousness. We need to realize that thoughts and emotions manifest in our body, and that when we know ourselves, we help ourselves to heal, to care, to love, to recognize that we are holistic beings (body, mind and spirit).

Although I have kept this story true to her words, I have removed certain parts of her testimonial where she shows immense gratitude and thanks me for all of it. I felt a little uncomfortable including that part because I was only a channel through which SHE found the solutions and decided to make changes in her life. She should be grateful to herself and to God who has made it all possible.

The most beautiful part of this chapter is the experiences lived by my client during her intrauterine life. She discovered moments of premature delivery as well as experience of rejection and being an unwanted baby, all of which formed the basis of a future tumour in her life. Although we had nine sessions to work through the anxieties and fears felt during her birth time, I have chosen to share the most important experiences so that they may help us to exchange a meaningful dialogue about intrauterine life. She describes the following experience of her birth time:

"...I am going down and I have a lot of anxiety to see what is out there and I am descending. There I hit on my forehead on the bone of my mother but this is not going to hurt me because I am going to live. There are some hands that pick me up. I came out. I am looking at my mother, she smiles at me...the doctor picks me up and cuts my umbilical cord. They carry me to my mother and she hugs me and puts me on her chest and says to me that I am going to be all right. As I was born before time they have to carry me... My mother hugs me tightly; how her hearts beats. I am out."

Continuing to work with later incidents in her adult life, she lived and processed this traumatic experience. She confronted those moments and once she found that she was all right now, she was ready to process more and take more awareness of malignant energies behind it.

"...Before coming out I was sweating a lot. I was bothered by the bad smell around me but now I like it. I feel her arm, the skin of my mother. I feel such great love. It's like at some moment I did not want to live but now yes, there is a Majestic Being to who I should be grateful for being here. There is a brilliant light. And I see this majestic man, he is there and he smiles and says, "You did it, you have lot to do, go ahead and trust in yourself." ...this is a light of so much force, energy and love that it fills me up. Nobody notices it and they remain engrossed in what they do. This light is so tranquil that my heart calms down. Now the doctor takes me to the incubator and they tell me that my mom is going to be with me, and then they put a tube into my mouth...Yucky...

In another session we continued to pick up more segments of that event and here that idea is to make visible which was invisible at that time for her.

"…When I was in the womb, I had a fear of taking birth because I did not know what was going to happen. My parents fight a lot and this scared me when I was in the womb. What for I am going to go out to this strange world if people shout. What I come here for… I was up there and I was very tranquil, lot of peace, so I did not understand that I had to be here. I wanted to go back but I could not, I did not want to come out because I was scared to be out and the same fear sometimes stopped me to take decisions and may be I get hurt, this is my insecurity, I did not trust on my decisions. When I was up there the master spoke a lot with me, when I came, I was not able to speak, communicate, ask, later when I grew up, I felt fear of asking and later I preferred listening, at some time I lost my confidence in myself and I did not trust what I was saying, sometimes I searched Master in different persons so that they can guide me. My Master is not here and I had to take my decisions… insecurity, not trusting myself. I should trust myself and also on the things I say, obviously, I am not going to hurt myself. I had fear of listening and speaking to myself…it is like I was incomplete but now I talk to myself and I am going to be completing myself like a piece was missing. I am complete with myself because I understand myself, I see myself as a dolphin (dolphin is a symbol of the power of regeneration) like I am doing therapy with myself…"

"… I was tired in the womb and decided to come out but then I got scared that I was still not complete (formed) and I had little more to go. Mom was telling that I have to have 9 months in order to be complete and I remembered that I was not formed and I could not go back and I thought if I go out incomplete then my Mom, Dad, siblings were not going to love me. It scared me and I feel it in my stomach and head. The same fear I feel when

I am up there and Master tells me to go to the earth and I say that I am not ready and there are things to learn and this is my family and they are going to reject me and he tells me that I have to go down. I go down but I do not like it... I do not want to be there so I went to conception...this is a very rare sensation that I had there and now understand why I felt incomplete but I have felt rejection. I do not accept myself...this big fear I had, unconsciously I thought that people rejected me because I did not accept myself. When people came closer I made myself move away. It was with men because I was annoyed with my Master and I rejected men in my life. I have been very hard on myself that is why I have always judged so much. On knowing and recognizing I am complete with myself. If I accept myself then I do not care if others do not accept me, it is like a wave which goes up and it is gone, like a life, goes up, comes down, good and bad moments. There is no fear but real acceptance (what a simple and profound statement!)... not only it happens to me but others too and this is how the life is and it happens to everyone. I had put myself on an electric chair and with every error I punished myself and now I understand that it is normal and I was defective and this is how we human beings are...

Then, she speaks to herself and this is a climactic moment as she begins to integrate the basic fears in her life, including the fear of not being fully formed. Her fear is being dissolved as she chooses to face reality.

"...You need to be calm and you should not be afraid of taking birth...I am a perfect being. People need 9 months to form but for me only 7. I am complete... there are many moments of happiness when you want to laugh and there are moments of sadness and this is the lesson of life...I mess up, I fall down and this is alright. When you learn to walk, at first you fall down and then get up and carry on. Life has lot of love for me...now I feel calmer and I am going to take birth but not with fear. My heart is now

softer (heart beats calmly and she laughs a little)…I am curious to come out…

After understanding and processing that anxiety at the moment of birth, she re-lives the natural process of her birth and has full awareness of coming out of complete hypnosis:

"…I am curious to come out of this thing like a tunnel which has a bone and at the end there is a hole from where I am going to go out. I feel so special and there is a mixture of emotions… and there is a man who is talking to me…they cut my umbilical cord, now they take me to clean because I am little bit dirty with blood and my mother moves her arm towards me and they take me away and I am calm…Life.

You can see for yourself that she is discovering herself; but here comes another important part where she discovers and processes the cause of her tumour more in detail. The session started with same moments of birth to resolve the remaining anxieties connected to her suicide attempt while in the womb:

"…It hurts, I am coming out… it is true that I do not want to come out because I am still not complete. Mom discussed with the Doctor and I still do not have 9 months, I want to go back, my mother pushes me and I do not want and I slip in this water… gelatin, I try to go back and I move a lot. I see a light outside and I hit and I hit with a bone and my forehead hurts a lot and lots of things are coming…I feel little doubtful, Mom, Dad, Siblings get scared and they reject me but a voice tells me that I am completely formed and this is my great master from up there enters and he says that I am complete and this gives me the security of coming out. I am out and this part hurts me a lot (points at the part of her forehead where she had a tumor) and this is my feminine side that I hit…it is a fear that I am incomplete and that something is not alright, I lack an ear, a shoulder then they are going to reject me, this is how they are speaking and this is my fear. When I became

very frightened I wanted to kill myself …they would not accept me because I am not fully formed…"

As an adult, this intrauterine experience turned into a benign tumor in her pituitary gland. Later in a session, she understood that her mother never rejected her; in fact, she loved her. One of the biggest discoveries she had was to realize that everything her mother felt was transmitted to her and that it was not her fear but her mother's fear that blocked her in life and created barriers to her freedom to enjoy. She covered herself with the blanket of fear, an emotion her mother created. Likewise, this is something her mother also received from her mother who received from hers and so on.

We need to reflect and understand the deeper meaning underlying this pattern. We were born to belong to our family through good, healthy connections and not through pathological ones but either way we are connected. I do not know whether it is true or not – perhaps I am entirely wrong in this-- but I have discussed it here and now it is up to you to accept or reject it. If you are told that your father has diabetes and your mother does as well, then you could have it too. Does it mean that unconsciously you created circumstances in your life that will lead you to develop diabetes because it is your unconscious way of relating with your family, and proving your loyalty or sense of belongingness to them?

The best any therapist can do to heal is "Love."
Atul Mehra

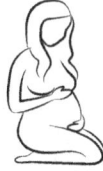

Chapter 10

More Intrauterine Mysteries Revealed

By adding this final chapter I wish to describe some more experiences detailing how a baby feels inside his mother's womb. I just thought to add some of my clients' experiences who have graciously allowed me to share them with my readers. They are very brave to make that decision, as most people would feel too uncomfortable to talk about it. I am deeply grateful to them for their valuable contribution. I will simply write down the experiences as they occurred in the mother's womb without providing an interpretation or analysis. I think that now after reading all these chapters you have sufficient experience and knowledge to understand it and conclude for yourself.

The first case is connected to Gaby who began her sessions with me some time ago. I had decided to write how she felt before and after the sessions because the lessons she learnt in her life have helped me understand many things. Moreover, many of us would identify with those conditions because we all have had similar experiences as human beings. These experiences become a beacon of light in the darkness as they guide us to understand our experiences so that we may learn to grow through them. This is what makes us feel that our past unfortunate experiences were necessary because we are meant to accept and learn from them. Neither can we change our history nor can we alter the course of events that led to our present state because it was the only path, so accepting and making peace with our past becomes an imperative goal in our life. Hope is a powerful force that sustains us through life and keeps us grounded in the face of an uncertain and unknown future. If we knew what future holds for us then there would be no need for hope. This is why life is so dynamic and wonderful.

Gaby started her session when she was 26 years old. Her therapeutic process lasted for two years, and here I provide an account of the experiences she felt.

It was a difficult decision for me to undergo therapy because I was very skeptical and closed, and furthermore it was scary to face my past. One day, as fate would have it, I went to his office, we talked and I realized that it was time to do something for myself, and I started my therapy. It was a great but a very difficult experience. I continued my therapy, but very often I looked for excuses to leave it. At first, I started to believe that it was all a figment of my imagination, but gradually I understood that he was bringing up my old shut off memories. First of all, I found myself in therapy realizing that there was someone different projecting inside me because many fears and fantasies controlled me. These fears did not belong to me because they were passed on to me by my mother. I gradually felt more confidence in myself and therapy became a time to relax and I began to listen and understand myself.

The best part of therapy was when I went through those sessions in the mother's womb, the experience of returning to this space, contact with my mother and to understand how I was being formed. All these experiences have been very valuable to me. The contact and connection with my inner child is also helping me a lot in every moment of my life. Before this, I was very timid and fearful. I allowed myself to be easily dominated by others. Now, little by little, I have felt more security in myself, and I became aware that it was time to live and to do the things I can do. The increased confidence in myself makes me do things which I once thought would be impossible to do, but now I have done all of that and with very little effort. Thanks to this therapy, I cured some ailments like allergies (especially to metal), and I have controlled my anxiety for sweets. I was not aware that I had reactions such as harming my skin by scratching or pulling my hair, but now I do not do it anymore. Now, I am 30 years old and I cannot say that generally my life has changed; I simply see it with different eyes. The change has occurred in me and now I enjoy every moment. I always repeat that I am a complete human being. I do not need anybody and I can do anything if I believe in myself."

Birth Time

I feel good, curious, I hear lots of voices. My mom says that time has come. There are unknown voices and the only known one is the doctor of my mother. She is calm and I am curious as to who these people are. I feel a lot of warmth...I feel internal warmth, I listen to my mother, my siblings and I feel curious. I have to take a breath...that I should be calm...my mother says that I have to breathe. There is a small moment when my mother gets scared and others too that I am not breathing but I take a breath at the time of birth, and that was not the time (to breathe) but I am calm and my mother too. (Now she goes to the moments when her mother feels scared so that part can be understood and integrated) *Mom is scared and I do not understand what is happening…my Mother feels scared and it worries me a little bit…I stop breathing and it amuses me because I know that I can handle that. It was not anything abnormal but it provoked anxiety. I feel a bit confused because I do not understand and I feel anxiety in my stomach.*

Birth time (2nd session)

I have to confront this fear from my mother that she is not able to protect me. I feel that if I stop breathing, she loses control of what happens to me. This is her fear and I need independence. I do not depend anymore on her and this is a separation…it is not easy but it has to happen. I have always realized that my mother worries about me, sometimes I feel worried when it comes to protection and it starts to suffocate me. Generally she is with me, together and I need to be released so that I can breathe little bit… (Now she understands the root cause hiding beneath her mother's fear). *She (my mother) feels two things: first, she is an adult woman and cannot take care of the girl and secondly, this is the fear she is holding from her past experience and she lived with my older sister* (during her birth time) *and this experience she had to live again. If not she would be more relaxed and calmer and I could confront it. This is not my fear and I should feel calm. It is understandable that I should feel that I should be born peacefully and I am going to transmit this tranquillity to her. She is calm…free from this responsibility…I feel calm, happy and I like what I am living. I feel freedom.*

Birth time (3rd session)

I am still in the belly of my mother and I feel good. (She goes into future and lives her after birth experience) *I am lying down in the cradle at the side of my mother; my mother is by my side and my siblings.* (Goes again into the future and remembers)…*the nurse and I are in the baby's room. There is no one I know but still I feel calm. I perceive things that I did not know before. Who are those voices that are around me and I want to be familiar with? My mother is in other room but I am calm.*

9th Month (Intrauterine life)

I feel very good, I am comfortable, I realize that I have grown; I hear a lot from my mother that my time for taking birth has come. I like to put my finger into the mouth. I can move my hands and feet, I can put my big toe…I like to investigate, it is a pleasant sensation on my face and to be able to feel myself, taste my finger and I feel these sensations in my stomach (although she finds it enjoyable but I observed that there is something she is hiding underneath and she brings up the memories of previous months to understand and resolve it). *I am 5 months old in my mother's womb; I realize that I have body parts. I listen to my mother say that she relishes when she is near me and she is mine and I am curious to know her.* (She discovers a connection and brings up the memories of 2nd month in her mother's womb). *I am almost 2 months old when my mother says that I am pregnant because she now knows that I exist. At last I can feel people come closer so that they can know that I am there. My mother puts her hand on her stomach and I feel her hug me and I want to hug her back but I do not have hands; she tells me that I am going to grow, and I am anxious to know how I am being developed. I have a lot of curiosity, there are many people speaking about me, how I am. I am going to have a surprise or this is really who I am. This is the sensation of independence. I am a complete self-sufficient being.* (The session ended so that next week we could probe the connection between anxiety and her adult life and she discovers something important).

9th Month continued

The connection with my body, putting fingers into my mouth, this anxiety comes from my mother, when she felt the need for protection, she would eat and this is my form of putting finger into my mouth. With this anxiety I put my finger into my mouth. I picked one of her forms to escape and converted it into mine. Many times I felt fear. Instead of speaking out, I put my finger into my mouth and shut my mouth. I always found something to hide and I chose to feel anxiety, which was not mine.

I put my finger into my mouth because I want to be with my mother. When she eats, she feels calm. When I feel her stressed, I feel that too and I put my finger into my mouth; but this fear does not belong to me…it is her who feels scared, not me. I should speak up about how I feel and not to be quiet or hide myself into the food. I know I always sucked my finger when I sometimes felt lonely, but now I understand why I do that. I used to look at it as fun that was not for me but for my Mom. If I keep on doing it then it is not going to be good for me. I feel calm. I can speak. When I put my finger into my mouth, I can't. Now I can do it peacefully and I am knowing myself.

8th Month (Intrauterine life)

I feel very good, comfortable. I can feel that there is a great deal of happiness around me, I can move and I know that I am being observed when my mother goes to the doctor and he examines me. I feel that I have a connection with others. I am not the one who they listen to but others can see me too. I feel a connection.

7th Month

I feel very good, I am very comfortable; above all, I listen to my mother singing, she knows when I move. She is always happy...well...I also feel happy. My father is near me and he likes to touch my mother's belly. I feel excited and I feel a kind of warmth every time the hand comes closer, I hug, I feel a lot of warmth...I move...I feel free, I can move, I can change different positions and I can play...movement.

6th Month

I feel good, comfortable with the place where I am, I like what surrounds my mother, many people talk, and I feel my mother is very calm, very happy. I feel the same with whatever I hear and very free...I feel complete and lots of excitement. I have so many parts (body) and they all belong to me...I am recognizing myself.

5th Month

I feel good at the place I am...this is the space where I can move with more freedom and I have more contact with people, they are out there...my mother and my father.

4th Month

I feel a bit uneasy, I want to move, the space does not allow me to move a lot, I feel my mother like I am growing up fast and she tells me to stay still and this bothers her because I make her feel uncomfortable and I feel these sensations in my stomach. (She brings up the memory of her 3rd day after conception in her mother's womb). *I am barely 3 days old in my mother's womb and I feel that I am in a very tight space and I try to express that I am there, I have arrived but there is no way I can communicate with my mother. She says that she feels bad...at the moment when I want to talk to her she feels bad and it makes me feel uneasy.*

It is to understand that at one moment it could affect others and in a certain way it was hurting because I felt bad and that's why I don't act so that others do not feel bad...it is a fear...feeling dependent on others, sometimes I stop doing things that are good for me. I have created a dependency of what others think of me. I should be sure of what I do. I should give up the sensations of feeling bad for others...not to feel responsible for other person...at some moment I believed that I was affecting my mother and I heard that she felt bad and I thought it was because of me...but the ravages (of pregnancy) *she felt were natural that occurred in her body but I felt that I was responsible...but I realize that I am not responsible for that. It does not mean that I do not love her...*(and now she discovers something very deep)... *when my mother got pregnant, she was scared because her older son was also going to be a father and she was also showing pregnancy symptoms and she was not able to deal with it.* (Now the integration happens because things are clearer and more visible; she feels the true desires of her mother towards her). *These uneasy sensations are not mine, my mother wants me to grow fast and I also want to grow fast to be able to be with her, so that she does not feel ravages anymore...so I should grow and I am being developed and she is happy that I grow up well...I do not have responsibility of what is happening, simply it is something natural that has to happen...freedom.*

3rd Month

I feel good, very comfortable, and very happy, everybody knows that I am here...I wanted them to know that how I took awareness that I am here and they know that I am here...I feel it like a strong connection with my mother, she is always loving me and taking care of me...always...I feel like lots of warmth around me...connection.

2nd Month

I feel very well, I am trying to know what is around me, I feel and listen to many things because I feel through my mother, I can get familiar with many things, she like to teach and I like to learn...because I am very curious...I want to know everything and I feel that she understands me...knowing.

1st Month

I feel happy and I feel that my mother feels that I am here... in spite of the fact that she is nervous, she feels happy. I feel this is something that does not depend on me because she does not know what is happening in her body...it gives me lots of curiosity, I feel excited and I feel it in my stomach.

She takes awareness.

At some moment I felt nervous same as she (mother) felt, fear of something completely new...one always tends to feel nervous about something that he does not know...I hope that it is going to be exciting and she has to take it easy, maybe these fears and nervousness take control and not allow to see the positive side. I understand that my mother feels nervous and fearful that a change is about to happen, maybe to her body or having a daughter, but always there is something to learn...I hope...like I learn...at some moment I felt her nervousness and I want to return it to you and I want to receive good...every moment there are changes so for that reason one has to learn in order to grow. Continue with these desires to know everything you want...I feel lots of love, very calm...change."

Sperm Consciousness

I am at a very clear place. I want to arrive someplace and I am moving very fast and it is very enjoyable to be able to

> *move in many different places...there is lots of light,*
> *emotion... a sound of laughter which comes from somewhere*
> *inside, very happy, it is accompanied by lots of light and vivid*
> *colors that ignite...I reach a very big light...this light enters*
> *and it is like something exploded, lots of lights turn on and*
> *lots of colours scatter happiness around me. Lots of light*
> *enters and moves in circles like a lot of water...I feel that I*
> *start to take a form, more defined...like I start to grow bigger*
> *by taking a more definite shape, to be able to stretch and to*
> *be able to touch...there is an ovum and I enter there...I begin*
> *to combine with it and a light enters. I feel good...growing."*

The Second Case

Jenny came to me when she was 21 years old. During her therapeutic process she discovered a powerful reason for her premature birth. She discovered that her mother used to feel alone and she wanted her daughter to be with her, so this caused a premature delivery that resulted in her taking birth. I decided to add some of her intrauterine experiences, as there are different reasons to see and understand for premature delivery.

Birth time (7th month)

I needed to come out; I did not want to be with my mother.
I do not want to be with my mother, she is very worried,
anxious. My father makes her feel bad and he is worried too,
I feel guilty and I feel these sensations in my stomach (she
brings up a memory of 5th and 3rd month of her intrauterine
life). *I am 5 months old and my mom is very worried and*
disturbed because of a decision she has to take with my
father... I feel bad because I have something to do with it. (In
the same session now she also recollects when she is 3 months

old in mother's womb). *I am with my mother and I am 3 months old and I am going to be a burden...my brother is sick...I wanted to come out so that I don't feel guilt and burden...I feel like that, because I do not know what is happening... like I am with my mother, I feel responsible of the quarrel. I felt responsible and part of the quarrel but I can detach myself from that. I am not responsible and I have got nothing to do with the problems of my parents. I cannot let myself get affected by others' words because they can make me feel bad I need to learn to value myself and I need to free myself from this...I feel calm, more* free (she moves and this is sense of movement). *I feel acceptance and I feel more calm...freedom.*

6th month (Intrauterine life)

I feel that I need to go out. I don't want to be with my mother, she is very worried and agitated, I cannot be with her anymore and I feel these sensations in my stomach... I am 3 or 4 months old (in womb) and I feel that I am going to be a burden. I feel like a burden... I am 2 months old (in womb). My mother is busy with Pablo (older brother)... she has to do her therapies, it does not make me feel bad but my mother is tired. I do not want to share this sentiment, physical tiredness, problems. I am a separate person and I have a right to feel my own sentiments because it is natural.

She further reflects: *Everyone is responsible for his or her own emotions; I cannot take care of her problems. It is true that I worry more and give priority to other person first, may be it is a support for other person but do not involve me, I have always thought that my mother would not be happy but it is not in my* hand (she processes that statement)...*less worried and more free. She loves me a lot. I feel good, warmth, protected and I am good with myself and I know myself.*

5th month

Now arriving on 5th month she experiences calmness as she has already taken awareness and integrated that part in one of the previous sessions.

I feel good, everything is all right, inside and outside, I am calm and content and I feel good.

4th month

"I feel good, my mother knows that I am going to be a daughter and she always wanted that, she accepts me and she waits for me, I do not know if I would contemplate her, in accompanying her that she dresses me and comb my hair… it makes me think what she expected…She thought that someone would think like her, she feels a little frustrated. I feel these sensations in my stomach."

(Due to some reasons I decided to continue only up to the 4th month of her intrauterine life)

The Third case

Roberto is a 20-year-old man who came because he felt that he was a kind of silent and introverted person who did not have a very good relationship with his family, especially his father. Although he did well academically, he was still not satisfied with his life and had issues with family relationships. The whole life therapy process took less time than expected as he resolved his problems faster and one of the main reason was that his mother comparatively lived a healthy pregnancy period. During his birth time he discovers the relationship with his senses and the sense of connection with the sense of telepathy. His father helps him to discover that hidden bond which was missing in his life and this bond is re-established. He lives and discovers some interesting awareness of himself in the 5th month inside his mother's womb.

Birth Time

I can feel that my all senses are very sharp...smell, touch, and hearing...I can feel that they are awake...as I can feel different textures, many new things I can feel, I listen to different sounds, different smells...I listen to different tone of voices like lot of noise, friction clothing...makes me feel very good... listening, touching, smelling.... I do not feel such an abrupt change in vision...it is something foggy...I feel more movement which catches my attention and touch...many persons are helping my mother and nearby I feel the presence of more mothers. My father is waiting for us...I feel lots of love as I am wrapped up as a part of my mother...my dad is far...they are certain of how I feel and they are certain of how I am. I feel bigger...it makes me feel myself...Feel.

9th Month (Intrauterine life)

I feel like I have a relationship with my family...a bond with everybody...they were preparing so that I would take birth... it makes me feel that I have a level of importance in my family...a place that is already marked...I feel quite protected...warmth.

8th Month

I feel calm...I believe that I am keep on knowing me...I try to close my eyes and...relaxed...I feel comfortable... satisfied...calmness.

7th Month

I feel excited...I am happy, I try to express it through movement...I believe that I am transmitting it to my mother...

it's awesome, she has work to do...I feel peace, I feel happy, that is why...it makes me feel excited...grace.

6th Month

I am concentrating...it's like I am taking idea of understanding my environment...I mean...my mother's environment...calm (mother)...it makes me feel a "connection" with my mother and in a certain way I perceive and learn from the energy which is around me...there is a sensation of warmth and cold...more sensation of being comfortable and less of being uneasy...sensation of being with myself and with other...I perceive the pleasure of feeling myself and with it I can receive and learn. It makes me feel that my body is a form of love...my own love...I feel complete...Recognition.

5th Month

I feel that I am sleepy, I feel little bit tired, I just want to take rest...sleep...I feel weak energy...it seems to me that may be my mom was emotionally disturbed and she has had more desire to put up with. I feel the lack of food. I believe that it is transmitted energy and I can perceive the energies and I started to feel like that...I feel many times what my mother feels, but I should tell her that I have to feel what I can feel and my mind, energy and body give the idea and tell me "this is not her fault, only I should start to differentiate, among my own sensations more than anything and to know that rest of them lack in myself (it is very important for a baby to feel himself and choose to connect with mother with healthy connections and not through depression, sadness etc. Can it change the dynamic of present or future diseases or disorders?). He continues...

I feel that sometimes my mother has can precisely transmit certain sensations, she has also felt happy or sad...I do not want to be sad...I do not have to carry my parent's sensations...I can recognize my sensations. (The simple sensations felt in mother's womb can influence and decide baby's future). He continues to take awareness.

I should feel myself more...try to be in meditation only with myself and this is going to help me to feel what "I want". There is something bad I can feel and I should understand, the truth that I feel and I cannot let myself get affected by different people or energies...I should not try to exert my mother's pressure on me. I can be loving and she can too. I can be calm and now I do not want to sleep...I was not feeling my energies like I wanted to feel but I felt that I was receiving the energies of my mother and now consciously I can keep on feeling myself in calmness...Unique.

4th Month
I feel good, I feel how I am growing, I feel that she (mother) *is very tranquil and it makes me feel calm...connection.*

3rd Month
I feel good, I feel quite comfortable like I have space for everything because I can move. I feel the capacity...sensations of feeling free and I can move in any direction...I feel my mother is also calm...Space.

2nd Month
I feel pretty happy...I feel everybody in my family is there... in this way this emotion is like joy...happiness.

1st Month
I feel quite calm. I stay still...I feel like an emotion inside me...as if I am a part of everything...complete.

I hope all these experiences described in this chapter will help you to understand and reflect in a different way than before. I hope this awareness of intrauterine experiences answers many of your questions of curiosity. I also wish for each one of you to share his/her awareness and curiosity with others so that all of us can work to ensure healthy and prosperous pregnancies. Life must continue no matter what.

Conclusion

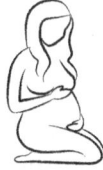

I am very happy to share all this information with you; together we have taken a step forward and I hope that many of you will continue moving forward. I hope that each and every one of you will be able to provide guidance to others for a healthy pregnancy should they opt to have a baby sometime in the future. Many of you may have found some personal connection to the information shared in this book and in your own lived experiences. I hope now that we have arrived at the end of this book, the baby's life in his mother's womb is no longer a mystery, and that most of you have accepted the fundamental idea of the perception and sensibility of the intrauterine life.

Many of you will agree that one of the most important things in life is to find inner freedom and balance in our world. The quest for self-transformation starts within; one of the most difficult steps – the first step – to take before anything else is to accept ourselves as we are. My journey began from the moment I heard my grandmother giving advice to my mom when she was pregnant with my little brother. Many years later, which included 17 years of practice and an abundance of curiosity, I found myself being propelled out of the traditional thought patterns and resistances. I had found progress at each stage of my development as my own thinking gradually evolved on this matter.

Our intrauterine life forms the foundation for the rest of our lives. A baby enjoys the privileges of being a super-conscious being: his connections with his mother through the 18 senses pre and post-birth directly or indirectly influence his life. His future is decided before birth and if he receives warmth, understanding and experiences of unconditional love and togetherness from his mom and dad, then he will live a happy and content life. He will have the ability to face life's challenges with calmness and wisdom. On the other hand, if he experiences rejection, doubt and incomprehension, he will live a life filled with sadness, pain, and unfulfilled potential. His capabilities will remain undeveloped and he will unfortunately suffer confusion and emptiness throughout his life. He might be "successful" in the eyes of society, but he will feel hollow inside.

I have conveyed my passions and convictions with all my heart and with a genuine simplicity. My hope is for all parents to continue helping their babies so that they may have the opportunity to live a healthy and fulfilling life. I leave you to reflect upon your own experiences in life and to find your own answers.

Until then, may every baby enjoy his birthright of unconditional love in and outside of his mother's womb!

References

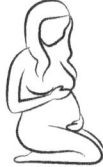

Anonymous. Article on Telepathy
http://www.themystica.com/mystica/articles/t/telepathy.html)
Cevallos, Diego (2008). Monografía, El Primer Botón [Monograph, The
   First Button], Quito, Ecuador
Dr. Lipton, Bruce (2005). The Biology of Belief, Publisher Hay House,
   18 Edition
Imbert, Claudia (2004). El futuro se decide antes de nacer [The future is
   decided before birth].
Editorial Desclee de Brouwer (Bilbao). Printed in Spain
Dr. Farrant, Graham (1988). An interview by Steven Raymond "Cellular
   consciousness and conception."
http://www.real-personal-growth.com/res_fixing/graham_farrant/
   graham_farrant_interview.htm
Herrera, Pablo (2005). Monografía, La unión psíquica niño-madre en
   la fase intrauterina desde el enfoque de la psicología profunda en
   Hipnosis [Monograph, The child-mother psychic union in the
   intrauterine phase from the deep psychology in Hipnosis
   Perspective]. Quito, Ecuador.
Jastrow, Robert (1981). Article, "Unlocking the Mysteries of the Mind,"
   The Tuscaloosa News, Dec, 6, 1981, Page 95 https://news.google.
   com/newspapers?nid=XUmZziuz7kC&dat=19811206&printsec=
   frontpage&hl=en
Jorge (2011). Comunidad Espiritual Virtual y Revista Digital Holistica
   [Virtual Spiritual Community and Holistic Digital Magazine].
   Article, Claves Para Vivir En Amor Incondicional De Los
   Hermanos Indios Hopi {Keys to Live Unconditional Love of the
   Indian Brothers Hopi]
http://hermandadblanca.org/claves-para-vivir-en-amor-incondicional-
   de-los-hermanos-indios-hopi/

135

Meinhold, Werner (2013). Introduction to Integrative depth psychology in therapy in research of analytical hypnosis. Koroni, Greece.

Meinhold, Werner (2008). El Gran Manual de la Hipnosis [The Great Manual of Hypnosis]. Editorial Trillas, Mexico, First Edition.

Meinhold, Werner (2010). Psicoterapia en Hipnosis [Psychotherapy in Hypnosis]. Editorial Trillas, Mexico.

Meinhold, Werner (2010). V Seminario Internacional de Terapia Integrativa de Psicología Profunda bajo Hipnosis [The 5th International seminar of Integrative therapy of depth Psychology in Hypnosis]. Quito, Ecuador.

Meinhold, Werner (2001). VI Seminario de la Hipnosis Terapéutica I.T.T.H. [The 6th Seminar of Therapeutic Hypnosis I.T.T.H.]. Quito, Ecuador.

Meinhold, Werner (2001). VII Seminario sobre Hipnosis Analítica de Psicología Profunda [The 7th Seminar on Analytical Hypnosis of Depth Psychology]. Quito, Ecuador.

Meinhold, Werner (2002). VIII Seminario de la Hipnosis Terapéutica I.T.T.H. [The 8th Seminar of Therapeutic Hypnosis I.T.T.H.]. Quito, Ecuador.

Meinhold, Werner (2003). X Seminario de la Hipnosis Terapéutica I.T.T.H. [The 10th Seminar of Therapeutic Hypnosis I.T.T.H.]. Quito, Ecuador.

Meinhold, Werner (2004). XI Seminario Internacional de Hipnología. [The 11th International Seminar on Hypnology]. Quito, Ecuador.

Meinhold, Werner (2005). XII Seminario Internacional de la Hipnosis Terapéutica I.T.T.H. [The 12th International Seminar of Therapeutic Hypnosis I.T.T.H.]. Quito, Ecuador.

Meinhold, Werner (2006). XIII Seminario Internacional "Reencarnación" [The 13th International Seminar on "Reincarnation"]. Quito, Ecuador.

Meinhold, Werner (2008). XVI Seminario Internacional de "Sexualidad" [The 16th International Seminar on "Sexuality"]. Quito, Ecuador.

Meinhold, Werner (2009). XVIII Seminario Internacional de "Cancer, Orígenes Emocionales, Prevención y Terapia bajo Hipnosis" [The 18th International Seminar on "Cancer, Emotional Origins, Prevention and Therapy in Hypnosis"]. Quito, Ecuador.

Meinhold, Werner (2010). XIX Seminario Internacional de Hipnosis "La conciencia humana" [The 19th International Seminar on "The Human Consciousness"]. Quito, Ecuador.

Meinhold, Werner (2010). XIX Seminario Internacional de Hipnosis "La conciencia humana" [The 19th International Seminar on "The Human Consciousness"]. Quito, Ecuador.

Pollan, Michael (2014). Article at www.pri.org "New research on plant intelligence may forever change how you think about plants." http://www.pri.org/stories/2014-01-09/new-research-plant-intelligence-may-forever-change-how-you-think-about-plants)

www.ingramcontent.com/pod-product-compliance
Lightning Source LLC
Chambersburg PA
CBHW050729030426
42336CB00012B/1475